Thriving Through Herbal Wisdom: A Bible of Natural Remedies

By Olivia Healinghart

Olivia Healinghart

Copyright © 2023 by Little Ink Publishing

Disclaimer:

The information presented in this book is intended for educational and informational purposes only. It is not intended as a substitute for professional medical advice, diagnosis, or treatment. Always seek the advice of your physician or other qualified healthcare provider with any questions you may have regarding a medical condition or the use of herbal remedies. The author and publisher of this book do not endorse any specific herbal remedies or treatments and disclaim any liability for any adverse effects resulting from the use of information provided herein. You should consult with a qualified healthcare professional before using any herbal remedies discussed in this book.

ISBN: 9798865487890

Table of Contents

Introduction

Welcome to a comprehensive guide designed to empower you with a profound understanding of the natural world's treasures. The following pages explore various natural remedies derived from plants, mushrooms, and trees. This book serves as your key to unlocking the vast potential of these resources, enriching your knowledge about their historical significance, scientifically proven applications, cultivation, harvesting, preservation, preparation techniques, recommended dosages, and potential interactions with conventional medicines. From tracing the footsteps of generations past and exploring how these natural remedies are trusted and embraced across diverse cultures, we transition to scientifically proven applications. Here, we bridge the past and present, delving into modern scientific research. You discover the medically proven benefits of these natural resources as we uncover their potential to address specific health conditions. Our approach remains firmly rooted in evidence and insight.

Turning our attention to the earth beneath our feet, we provide practical advice on cultivating these natural resources, whether it is in your backyard or within appropriate environments. You learn about soil conditions, planting zones, and the best times of the year for growth. Cultivation naturally leads to the act of gathering. We offer guidance on when to pluck the fruits of your labor. Timing is everything when it comes to maximizing the therapeutic potential of these natural resources. Nature's bounty is not always within arm's reach. We explore ways to ensure these remedies remain accessible, even out of season. You discover the art of drying, freezing, and other techniques that preserve their medicinal properties. With your harvest in hand, it is time to prepare the elixirs of well-being. The Medicinal Resources section outlines various methods for creating remedies. You learn how to make teas, tinctures, infusions, and topical applications, ensuring the full potential of each resource is made available. Safety is paramount, and recommended dosages guide you in responsibly using these natural remedies. We stress the importance of consulting healthcare providers or herbalists for personalized advice, ensuring your well-being. The purpose of this book is not to replace medical advice or necessary medications but to provide information on supplementing medical care with natural resources.

Lastly, we highlight the coexistence of natural remedies and conventional medicines. You discover the precautions to take and are encouraged to communicate with healthcare providers for seamless integration into your healthcare regimen. In addition to the knowledge presented in this guide, you also find an exciting bonus section, "Natural Recipes for Health." This segment takes your exploration of natural remedies to another level by showing you how to incorporate these resources into your daily life. You discover a range of delightful natural recipes that promote well-being and make the most of nature's offerings. From soothing teas and nourishing snacks to topical salves and tinctures, this bonus section lets you experience the therapeutic potential of these resources in the dishes and drinks you enjoy every day. Get ready to add a touch of nature's goodness to your daily meals. With this roadmap, we journey through the intricate world of health, medicinal resources, and herbal recipes, exploring their historical roots, modern applications, and practical implementation. Together, we embrace the wisdom of the natural world and enrich our lives with its treasures.

8

Health Topics

Acne

Acne is a common skin condition that occurs when hair follicles become clogged with oil, dead skin cells, and bacteria. Acne can affect various body parts but is commonly found on the face, neck, back, chest, and shoulders. It can occur at any age but is most common in adolescents and young adults.

Some natural remedies and skincare practices help manage and prevent acne or support skin health. These approaches should be used as complementary measures alongside evidence-based treatments. Some natural substances and methods explored for their potential benefit in managing acne include.

Tea Tree Oil (Melaleuca alternifolia). Tea tree oil, with its antibacterial and anti-inflammatory properties, can be use topically to help with acne. It should be diluted with a carrier oil to avoid skin irritation.

Aloe Vera (Aloe barbadensis miller): Aloe vera gel, known for its soothing and anti-inflammatory properties, may assist with skin healing and reduce redness associated with acne.

Honey: Honey, recognized for its antibacterial and wound-healing properties, can be applied in face masks or spot treatments.

Green Tea: Green tea, rich in antioxidants, can help reduce inflammation when applied topically or consumed as a beverage.

Witch Hazel: Witch hazel, possessing astringent properties, can serve as a natural toner to help control oil and reduce inflammation.

It is essential to consult a dermatologist or healthcare provider before starting any natural remedies to ensure they are safe and suitable for your skin type and condition. Skincare practices, such as using a gentle cleanser, avoiding excessive scrubbing, and selecting non-comedogenic (non-pore-clogging) skincare products, are essential for acne management. Natural remedies should be used under professional guidance and with prescribed acne treatments as needed.

Allergies

Allergies are immune system responses to substances that usually pose no harm but are perceived as threats by the body. These substances, known as allergens, trigger an allergic reaction when they encounter the body. Common allergens include pollen, dust mites, pet dander, certain foods, insect stings, and mold spores. Allergic reactions manifest in numerous ways, such as sneezing, a runny or stuffy nose, itchy or watery eyes, skin rashes, hives, and, in severe cases, anaphylaxis, a life-threatening reaction.

The primary allergy treatment typically involves allergen avoidance, medications, and, in some instances, allergen immunotherapy (allergy shots or sublingual tablets).

Medicines like antihistamines, decongestants, and corticosteroids help alleviate allergy symptoms. Additionally, certain lifestyle adjustments, like using air purifiers and maintaining a clean-living environment, reduce exposure to allergens.

While their effectiveness varies from person to person, and individual responses may differ, here are some examples of natural remedies that demonstrate potential in managing allergies:

Butterbur (Petasites hybridus): Butterbur is an herb studied for its potential benefit in relieving hay fever symptoms. Available in supplement form, it should be used as directed by a healthcare provider.

Quercetin: Quercetin, a flavonoid found in certain foods (e.g., apples, onions) and available in supplement form, possesses antioxidant and anti-inflammatory properties that may assist with allergy symptoms.

Stinging Nettle (Urtica dioica): Stinging nettle supplements may exhibit antihistamine and anti-inflammatory effects, potentially relieving allergy symptoms. They should be used as directed by a healthcare provider.

It is crucial to consult with a healthcare provider before starting any natural remedies, as their effectiveness and safety can vary among individuals. Allergy management should primarily involve allergen avoidance and, when necessary, prescribed medications. Natural remedies should serve as complementary measures to support overall allergy management. In cases of severe allergies or anaphylaxis, emergency medical care is necessary.

Alzheimer's Disease

Alzheimer's is a progressive neurodegenerative disorder that primarily affects the brain, leading to cognitive and functional decline. It remains the most common cause of dementia among older adults. Alzheimer's characterizes itself by accumulating abnormal protein deposits in the brain, including beta-amyloid plaques and tau tangles, which disrupt communication between brain cells and cause cell death.

The hallmark symptoms of Alzheimer's include memory loss, impaired thinking and reasoning, difficulty with problem-solving, and changes in behavior and personality. Individuals may have trouble performing everyday tasks and communicating as the disease progresses.

Currently, no cure exists for Alzheimer's, and the primary treatment focuses on managing symptoms and improving the individual's quality of life. Treatment may involve medication, cognitive and behavioral interventions, and support from healthcare professionals and caregivers.

Some natural remedies and dietary considerations are being explored for their potential benefit in supporting brain health and cognitive function. Discuss these approaches with healthcare providers and use them as complementary measures alongside evidence-based treatments for Alzheimer's. Here are a few natural substances that show promise in Alzheimer's research:

Ginkgo Biloba (Ginkgo biloba): Ginkgo biloba is an herb explored for its potential to improve cognitive function. It is available in supplement form, but its use should be discussed with a healthcare provider.

Turmeric (Curcuma longa): Curcumin, a compound in turmeric, has anti-inflammatory and antioxidant properties and may hold potential benefits for brain health. Add it to food or take it in supplement form.

Omega-3 Fatty Acids: Omega-3 supplements, particularly those containing eicosapentaenoic acid (EPA) and docosahexaenoic acid (DHA), are studied for their potential benefit in cognitive health. The appropriate dosage should be discussed with a healthcare provider.

Vitamin E: Vitamin E, an antioxidant, may support brain health. It can be obtained through dietary sources or supplements, but usage should be discussed with a healthcare provider.

It is essential to consult with a healthcare provider before starting any natural remedies, as their effectiveness and safety can vary among individuals. Alzheimer's is a complex condition, and it requires a comprehensive approach to treatment. Natural remedies should serve as complementary measures to support overall Alzheimer's Disease management and should not replace prescribed medications or evidence-based treatments. Regular follow-up with healthcare providers is crucial for monitoring the condition and adjusting treatment as needed.

Anemia

Anemia is a medical condition characterized by a deficiency in the number of red blood cells or a decrease in hemoglobin in the blood. Hemoglobin is a protein in red blood cells that binds to oxygen, enabling these cells to carry oxygen from the lungs to the rest of the body. Anemia can result in reduced oxygen delivery to tissues and organs, leading to symptoms such as fatigue, weakness, pale skin, shortness of breath, and cold hands and feet.

The treatment for anemia depends on its underlying cause, which can vary widely. Common causes of anemia include nutritional deficiencies (e.g., iron deficiency anemia), chronic diseases, genetic conditions, and bone marrow disorders. Treatment may involve addressing the underlying cause, making dietary changes, and, in some cases, supplementation with iron, vitamin B12, or other nutrients.

Some natural remedies and dietary considerations may help support individuals with anemia or low iron levels. Discuss these approaches with healthcare providers and use them as complementary measures to prescribed treatments. Some natural substances and foods explored for their potential benefit in managing anemia or improving iron levels include.

Vitamin C: Vitamin C enhances the absorption of nonheme iron (the type of iron found in plant-based foods). Consuming vitamin C-rich foods, like citrus fruits, berries, and bell peppers, alongside iron-rich foods can help improve iron absorption.

Nettle (Urtica dioica): Nettle leaves have been traditionally used to improve iron levels. Nettle tea or supplements may be considered.

Yellow Dock (Rumex crispus): Yellow dock root is known for its potential iron-enhancing properties. It can be consumed as tea or taken in supplement form.

Dandelion (Taraxacum officinale): Dandelion greens are a source of vitamins and minerals, including iron. They can be consumed in salads or cooked as greens.

It is important to consult with a healthcare provider to determine the underlying cause of anemia and receive appropriate treatment. Natural remedies and dietary changes should be made under professional guidance to ensure they are safe and appropriate for the individual's condition.

Anxiety and Stress

Anxiety and stress are prevalent experiences that can benefit from a comprehensive approach to management. While medicinal plants and other natural remedies might provide complementary support, they should not replace professional medical advice or treatments. Consulting with a healthcare professional for a comprehensive strategy is crucial. Several natural substances and practices have shown potential in assisting with anxiety and stress management:

Anxiety and stress, common emotional and physiological reactions to difficult or intimidating scenarios, are components of the body's innate "fight or flight" mechanism, aiding in our response to stressors. However, these feelings can adversely impact mental and physical well-being if they become persistent or overwhelming.

Anxiety manifests as discomfort, nervousness, or concern, frequently about forthcoming events or circumstances. It can produce physical symptoms like restlessness, muscle tightness, and constant thoughts. Various anxiety disorders, including generalized anxiety disorder, panic disorder, and social anxiety disorder, consist of intense and extended anxiety disrupting daily functioning.

Stress, a reaction to external strain or demands, typically arises concerning actual or perceived dangers. It can stem from multiple sources, such as work, personal relationships, financial issues, or significant life transitions. It can result in psychological and physical symptoms like tension, irritability, and sleep issues.

Some natural substances and activities have demonstrated potential in aiding the management of anxiety and stress:

Chamomile (Matricaria chamomilla): Chamomile, recognized for its tranquilizing and relaxing qualities, can be ingested as tea, or used as a supplement.

Lavender (Lavandula angustifolia): in the form of essential oil or tea, it might possess calming properties

Valerian (Valeriana officinalis): Valerian, potentially beneficial for relaxation and sleep, is accessible as a supplement or tea.

Exercise:
Consistent physical activity can diminish stress and anxiety levels by releasing endorphins and enhancing overall health.

Before initiating any natural remedies or practices, it is imperative to seek advice from a healthcare professional, as the efficacy and safety of these methods can differ significantly among individuals. Natural remedies should complement, not replace, scientifically supported treatments for anxiety and stress. A healthcare provider can offer guidance on the most suitable methods based on an individual's needs and symptoms.

Anxiety Disorders

Anxiety disorders comprise a set of mental health diagnoses defined by excessive, enduring worry, fear, or anxiety about various life situations. These disorders can notably disrupt everyday life and overall well-being. Common anxiety disorders include generalized anxiety disorder (GAD), panic disorder, social anxiety disorder, and specific phobias.

Several natural substances have undergone research for their potential benefits in easing anxiety symptoms, such as

Chamomile (Matricaria chamomilla): Chamomile, an herb celebrated for its tranquilizing and soothing qualities, can be drunk as tea, or administered as a supplement.

Valerian (Valeriana officinalis): Valerian, reputed for aiding in relaxation and sleep, is accessible as a supplement and tea.

Passionflower (Passiflora incarnata): Passionflower, researched for its potential sedative properties, might be obtainable in supplement form.

Kava (Piper methysticum): Kava, recognized for its anxiolytic (anxiety-relieving) effects, may be consumed traditionally as a drink in certain areas or as a supplement.

Lavender (Lavandula angustifolia): In the form of essential oil or tea, lavender may provide calming sensations.

It is vital to acknowledge that the effectiveness of these natural interventions can differ from person to person, and they should be approached with prudence. Anxiety disorders are multifaceted and managing them might necessitate a multifaceted strategy. These natural remedies should be considered as supplementary to overall anxiety treatment plans and discussed with healthcare professionals. The cornerstone of anxiety disorder treatment remains medications and psychotherapy, with healthcare professionals guiding toward the most fitting treatment choices based on an individual's unique requirements and symptoms.

Arthritis

Arthritis encompasses various conditions involving joint inflammation, leading to pain, stiffness, and swelling symptoms. Numerous types of arthritis exist, but osteoarthritis and rheumatoid arthritis are the most prevalent.

Osteoarthritis: This widespread form of arthritis appears with aging. It is a degenerative disease affecting joint cartilage and underlying bone, leading to their breakdown.

Rheumatoid Arthritis is an autoimmune disorder where the immune system erroneously targets the joints, prompting inflammation and subsequent damage.

While arthritis remains incurable, treatments focus on symptom management, pain reduction, and enhancing joint functionality. Typical treatment methods encompass medications, physical therapy, and lifestyle adaptations, with joint replacement surgery as a potential option in advanced cases.

Specific natural remedies and dietary adjustments are under investigation for their potential advantages in alleviating arthritis symptoms, including

Turmeric (Curcuma longa): Turmeric is known for its curcumin content and boasts anti-inflammatory qualities. It can be incorporated into meals or ingested as a supplement, though the proper dosage should be clarified with a healthcare provider.

Ginger (Zingiber officinale): With its anti-inflammatory features, ginger might assist in diminishing pain and inflammation associated with arthritis. It can be enjoyed as ginger tea or used in cooking.

Green Tea (Camellia sinensis): Abundant in antioxidants, green tea could offer anti-inflammatory benefits. It is commonly consumed as a drink.

Omega-3 Fatty Acids: Specific omega-3 fatty acids, especially eicosapentaenoic acid (EPA) and docosahexaenoic acid (DHA), are under study for their potential to curb arthritis-induced inflammation. An appropriate dosage should be determined with a healthcare provider.

Devil's Claw (Harpagophytum procumbens): This herb is studied for its potential to ease arthritis-related discomfort. Available as a supplement, the correct dosage should be confirmed with a healthcare provider.

Before initiating any natural remedies, seeking advice from a healthcare provider is imperative, as individual responses and safety considerations may differ. While prescribed medications and therapies remain the central strategy for arthritis management, natural remedies could serve as supplementary measures, supporting comprehensive arthritis care. Consistent check-ins with healthcare providers are vital for ongoing condition monitoring and necessary treatment adjustments.

Asthma

Asthma is a long-term lung disorder marked by airway inflammation and constriction, complicating breathing. Asthmatics commonly experience wheezing, coughing, a feeling of chest constriction, and breathlessness. The severity of asthma symptoms varies, with triggers including allergens, respiratory infections, physical activity, and environmental pollutants.

Standard asthma treatments primarily use medications like bronchodilators and corticosteroids to mitigate inflammation and facilitate airway opening. Healthcare professionals prescribe these based on the asthma's severity.

Natural remedies may serve as adjunctive support in asthma management but must not replace prescribed medications and should be vetted by healthcare professionals. Several natural substances are being explored for their potential asthma-relieving properties:

Butterbur (Petasites hybridus): This herb, potentially anti-inflammatory, might aid in managing bronchial asthma. Available as a supplement, it must be used under healthcare provider guidance.

Honey:
Traditionally used for its possible calming effect on the throat and helpfulness in asthma-related coughs, honey can be taken directly or mixed into warm liquids.

Ginger (Zingiber officinale): Known for its anti-inflammatory effects, ginger might assist with asthma symptoms. It is consumable as tea or used in meals.

Coffee:
Its caffeine content, a bronchodilator, could offer temporary asthma symptom relief. However, coffee consumption needs careful consideration, with a healthcare professional discussing specifics on quantity and timing.

Garlic (Allium sativum): Renowned for anti-inflammatory and immune-enhancing qualities, garlic is a beneficial dietary addition.

Recognizing that natural remedies' effectiveness can differ individually is crucial and should be approached cautiously. Asthma, a significant health concern, primarily depends on prescribed medications for management. Any supplementary methods need healthcare provider approval to confirm safety and suitability for the person living with asthma.

Attention-Deficit/Hyperactivity Disorder (ADHD)

Attention-Deficit/Hyperactivity Disorder (ADHD) is a neurodevelopmental disorder affecting children and adults. It is characterized by persistent inattention, hyperactivity, and impulsive patterns that can interfere with daily functioning and quality of life. ADHD typically gets diagnosed based on specific criteria, and it can manifest in several ways, with three primary subtypes:

Predominantly Inattentive Presentation: Individuals with this subtype have trouble sustaining attention, following through on tasks, and organizing activities.

Predominantly Hyperactive-Impulsive Presentation: Individuals with this subtype exhibit elevated levels of hyperactivity and impulsivity but might not necessarily have significant inattention.

Combined Presentation: Individuals with this subtype display a combination of inattention, hyperactivity, and impulsivity.

The primary treatment for ADHD involves a multimodal approach, including

Medication: Stimulant medications like methylphenidate and amphetamine-based drugs commonly prescribed to manage ADHD. These medications work to improve focus, attention, and impulse control.

Behavioral Therapy: Behavioral interventions, including cognitive-behavioral therapy and psychoeducation, assist individuals in developing coping strategies and improving time management and organizational skills.

Educational Support: In school and work settings, accommodations, and support, such as Individualized Education Plans (IEPs) and 504 plans, assist individuals with ADHD in succeeding academically and professionally.

While no cure exists for ADHD, some individuals and families explore complementary and alternative approaches. It is crucial to note that these approaches should be discussed with healthcare providers and used with evidence-based treatments. Some natural remedies and dietary considerations being explored in the context of ADHD management include.

Omega-3 Fatty Acids: Some studies suggest that omega-3 fatty acids, especially those containing eicosapentaenoic acid (EPA) and docosahexaenoic acid (DHA), may have a beneficial effect on attention and focus. These can be obtained from fatty fish like salmon mackerel or through fish oil supplements. The appropriate dosage and use should be discussed with a healthcare provider.

Ginkgo Biloba (Ginkgo biloba): Ginkgo biloba is an herb studied for its potential effects on cognitive function. Some individuals with ADHD explore ginkgo biloba supplements. However, their use should be discussed with a healthcare provider, and research on its effectiveness continues.

Ginseng (Panax spp.): Ginseng, especially Panax ginseng, is under study for its potential cognitive-enhancing properties. Ginseng supplements are available, but their use should be discussed with a healthcare provider, as the research is inconclusive.

It is important to stress that the effectiveness of these natural substances in managing ADHD symptoms varies among individuals. They should be considered complementary measures and should not replace prescribed medications or evidence-based treatments for ADHD. Consulting with a healthcare provider, especially those specializing in ADHD, is essential for making informed decisions about treatment options.

Furthermore, natural remedies and dietary changes must be made carefully, as individual responses can vary, and some individuals may have sensitivities or allergies to certain substances. Any dietary adjustments or supplement use should be discussed with a healthcare provider to ensure they are safe and appropriate for the individual with ADHD.

Autism Spectrum Disorder (ASD)

Autism Spectrum Disorder (ASD) is a complex neurodevelopmental condition affecting social interaction, communication, and behavior. ASD is characterized by a wide range of symptoms and behaviors, referred to as a "spectrum" disorder. Individuals with ASD can have varying degrees of impairment, and each person's experience with autism is unique.

Common features of ASD may include:

Challenges with Social Interaction: Difficulty understanding and responding to social cues, making eye contact, and forming relationships.

Communication Difficulties: Delay in speech and language development, difficulty with conversation, and reliance on nonverbal communication.

Repetitive Behaviors: Engagement in repetitive movements or behaviors, such as hand-flapping, rocking, or a strong adherence to routines.

Sensory Sensitivities: Heightened sensitivity to sensory stimuli, such as light, sound, texture, and taste.

Narrow Interests: Intense focus on specific interests or topics. Impaired Social Imagination: Difficulty understanding and predicting the thoughts and actions of others.

While no known cure exists for ASD, various therapies and interventions are helping manage its symptoms and improve the quality of life for individuals with autism. These may include behavioral therapy, speech therapy, occupational therapy, and educational support.

Some individuals and families are exploring complementary and alternative approaches. These approaches should be discussed with healthcare providers and used with evidence-based treatments. Some natural remedies and dietary considerations being explored in the context of ASD management include:

Some supplements, such as omega-3 fatty acids, vitamin B6, and magnesium, are under study for their potential benefit in managing certain symptoms of ASD. Consulting a healthcare provider before starting any supplements is crucial.

Herbal Teas: Chamomile and lemon balm teas can be consumed for their calming properties. These should be given under the guidance of a healthcare provider.

It is crucial to emphasize that the effectiveness of these natural remedies varies from person to person, and they should always serve as complementary measures alongside evidence-based treatments for ASD. The primary approach to managing ASD typically involves individualized interventions and therapies tailored to the person's needs and strengths. Consulting with a healthcare provider, especially those specializing in autism, is essential for making informed decisions about treatment options.

Autoimmune Diseases

Autoimmune diseases constitute conditions where the immune system mistakenly attacks healthy cells and tissues. The primary treatment for autoimmune diseases typically involves immunosuppressive medications, anti-inflammatory drugs, and disease-specific therapies. However, some natural substances from medicinal plants, mushrooms, and trees may offer complementary support and help manage specific symptoms and aspects of autoimmune diseases. Here are a few natural remedies that show promise in providing supportive benefits for individuals with autoimmune diseases:

Autoimmune diseases form a broad category of disorders in which the immune system, responsible for protecting the body against harmful invaders like bacteria and viruses, mistakenly attacks the body's own healthy cells and tissues. This immune system dysfunction leads to inflammation and damage in various organs and systems, creating a wide range of autoimmune conditions.

Some common autoimmune diseases include Rheumatoid Arthritis: The immune system attacks the synovium, the lining of the membranes that surround the joints.

Lupus (Systemic Lupus Erythematosus): Lupus can cause inflammation in the joints, skin, kidneys, and other organs, affecting various body systems.

Multiple Sclerosis: The immune system damages the protective covering of nerve fibers in the central nervous system.

Type 1 Diabetes: The immune system destroys insulin-producing cells in the pancreas, leading to high blood sugar levels.

Celiac Disease: The immune system reacts to gluten ingestion, damaging the small intestine.

Hashimoto's Thyroiditis: The thyroid gland gets attacked, leading to hypothyroidism.

Psoriasis: The immune system triggers rapid skin cell growth, resulting in thick, red, and scaly patches on the skin.

Inflammatory Bowel Disease (IBD): Chronic digestive tract inflammation includes Crohn's disease and ulcerative colitis.

Here are a few natural remedies that show promise in providing supportive benefits for individuals with autoimmune diseases:

Turmeric (Curcuma longa) contains curcumin, known for its anti-inflammatory and immune-modulating properties. It can be added to food or taken as a supplement.

Ginger (Zingiber officinale): Ginger possesses anti-inflammatory properties and can be consumed in various forms, such as tea or as a spice in cooking.

Green Tea (Camellia sinensis): Green tea, rich in antioxidants, may assist with inflammation. It can be consumed as a beverage.

Reishi Mushroom (Ganoderma lucidum): Reishi mushrooms have immune-boosting properties and may be available as a supplement.

Astragalus (Astragalus membranaceus): Astragalus is used in traditional medicine to support the immune system and reduce inflammation. It can be consumed as a supplement or in tea.

Licorice Root (Glycyrrhiza glabra): Licorice root may assist with inflammation and immune modulation and can be brewed as a tea.

Echinacea (Echinacea purpurea): Echinacea, known for its immune-enhancing properties, can be consumed as a supplement or in tea.

It is important to note that these natural remedies should be used cautiously, and consultation with a healthcare professional is crucial when dealing with autoimmune diseases. The primary treatment for autoimmune diseases typically involves medications, such as immunosuppressants or anti-inflammatories, prescribed by healthcare providers to manage symptoms and slow disease progression.

Bacterial Infections

Bacterial infections occur when harmful bacteria invade the body and multiply within it. Bacteria are microorganisms present in the environment, and while many types are harmless or beneficial, some can cause infections and diseases in humans. Bacterial infections can happen in various body parts and may lead to a wide range of symptoms, from mild to severe.

It is important to note that bacterial infections are typically treated with antibiotics, which are medications specifically designed to kill or inhibit the growth of bacteria. Antibiotics should be prescribed by a healthcare professional based on the type of bacteria causing the infection and its sensitivity to specific antibiotics.

Some natural substances with potential antimicrobial properties are being studied:

Garlic (Allium sativum). Garlic possesses natural antibacterial properties and may help support the immune system. It can be consumed as part of the diet or in supplement form.

Honey: Honey has been used for its antibacterial properties for centuries and can be applied topically to wounds and minor skin infections.

Goldenseal (Hydrastis canadensis): Goldenseal contains berberine, a compound with antimicrobial properties. It is available as a supplement.

Tea Tree Oil (Melaleuca alternifolia): Tea tree oil possesses antimicrobial properties and can be applied topically to minor skin infections. It should be diluted with a carrier oil.

Manuka Honey: Manuka honey is known for its potent antibacterial properties and is sometimes used topically on wounds and minor infections.

Echinacea (Echinacea purpurea): Echinacea is an herb often used to support the immune system and may help the body fight off infections.

It is crucial to emphasize that while these natural substances may have antimicrobial properties, they are considered supportive measures rather than primary treatments for bacterial infections. If you suspect a bacterial infection, it is essential to consult with a healthcare professional for a proper diagnosis and treatment. Antibiotics are the primary method.

Bipolar Disorder

Bipolar Disorder is a complex mental health condition that requires careful management, often including mood-stabilizing medications, psychotherapy, and lifestyle adjustments. Natural substances are not primary treatments for bipolar disorder but may provide supportive benefits and help manage certain symptoms. Always consult with a healthcare professional for a comprehensive treatment plan tailored to your specific needs. Here are some natural remedies that show potential to provide supportive benefits for individuals with bipolar disorder:

St. John's Wort (Hypericum perforatum): St. John's Wort is an herb known for its potential antidepressant effects. It is typically available as an herbal supplement, and the dosage can vary. Consult with a healthcare provider for guidance.

Omega-3 Fatty Acids: Fish Oil (Omega-3 Fatty Acids), found in fish oil, may positively impact mood regulation, and may benefit people with bipolar disorder. Fish oil supplements can be considered, but the dosage should be discussed with a healthcare provider.

Saffron (Crocus sativus): Saffron is a spice that shows potential in improving mood and reducing symptoms of depression. It can be used in cooking or consumed as a saffron supplement, with the dosage recommended by a healthcare provider.

Rhodiola (Rhodiola rosea): Rhodiola Rosea is an adaptogen herb that may help improve mood, reduce fatigue, and enhance cognitive function. Rhodiola supplements are available, and the dosage may vary. Consult with a healthcare provider for guidance.

Maitake Mushrooms (Grifola frondosa): Maitake Mushrooms contain compounds that may have mood-regulating effects. Maitake supplements are available, and the dosage can vary. Consult with a healthcare provider for guidance.

It is crucial to emphasize that these natural remedies should only be considered complementary measures and should not replace prescribed medications or professional guidance for bipolar disorder. The treatment of bipolar disorder is typically complex and may require ongoing medical supervision and support. Individual responses to these remedies can vary, and their effectiveness may differ from person to person.

Bladder Disorders

Bladder disorders encompass a range of conditions that affect the urinary bladder, leading to various symptoms such as urinary urgency, frequency, incontinence, or discomfort. These conditions can result from infections, inflammation, structural abnormalities, or neurological issues. Common bladder disorders include urinary tract infections (UTIs), interstitial cystitis, and overactive bladder. Here are a few natural remedies that show potential to provide supportive benefits for individuals with bladder disorders:

Cranberry (Vaccinium macrocarpon): Cranberries are often used to help prevent and manage urinary tract infections (UTIs) by inhibiting the adherence of bacteria to the bladder wall.

Consuming unsweetened cranberry juice or cranberry supplements can be beneficial.

Dandelion (Taraxacum officinale): Dandelion leaf tea is a diuretic and may help with bladder function and urinary tract health.
Brew dandelion tea and consume it.

Marshmallow Root (Althaea officinalis): Marshmallow Root is known for its soothing and anti-inflammatory properties and may help with irritated bladder symptoms. Brew marshmallow root tea and consume it.

Chamomile (Matricaria chamomilla): Chamomile is often consumed for its calming and anti-inflammatory effects and may help with discomfort associated with bladder disorders. Drink chamomile tea to relieve symptoms.

Corn Silk (Zea mays): Corn Silk has diuretic properties and may help with bladder and urinary tract health. Brew cornsilk tea and consume it.

Uva Ursi (Arctostaphylos uva-ursi): Uva Ursi is sometimes used to support urinary tract health and help prevent UTIs. Take uva ursi supplements as directed.

Horsetail (Equisetum arvense): Horsetail is known for its diuretic and anti-inflammatory properties and may support bladder and urinary health. Brew horsetail tea and consume it.

Buchu (Agathosma betulina): Buchu is traditionally used for urinary tract health and may help with bladder symptoms. Brew buchu tea and consume it.

Nettle (Urtica dioica): Nettle is a diuretic and may support overall bladder and urinary tract function. Brew nettle tea and consume it.

Goldenseal (Hydrastis canadensis): Goldenseal contains berberine, which has antimicrobial properties and is used to prevent UTIs.

Bloating and Gas

Bloating and gas are common gastrointestinal symptoms that can cause discomfort and a feeling of fullness in the abdominal area. These symptoms can occur for assorted reasons, including swallowing air while eating, consuming gas-producing foods, or underlying digestive issues. While occasional bloating and gas are normal, chronic, or severe symptoms may indicate an underlying digestive problem. Here are a few natural remedies that show potential in providing relief:

Peppermint (Mentha × piperita): Peppermint tea or oil can help relax the gastrointestinal tract muscles, reducing bloating and gas.
Drink peppermint tea or inhale peppermint oil vapor.

Ginger (Zingiber officinale): Ginger is known for its anti-nausea and digestive properties and can help alleviate bloating and gas. Consume ginger tea or incorporate ginger into your diet.

Fennel (Foeniculum vulgare): Fennel seeds or tea can have carminative properties, helping to reduce gas and bloating. Chew fennel seeds or brew fennel tea and consume it.

Chamomile (Matricaria chamomilla): Chamomile tea has anti-inflammatory properties and can help soothe the digestive system, reducing bloating and gas. Drink chamomile tea to relieve symptoms.

Anise (Pimpinella anisum): Anise seeds can help digestion and reduce gas when consumed as a tea or a spice. Chew anise seeds or brew anise tea and consume it.

Caraway (Carum carvi): Caraway seeds can have carminative effects and can be used to reduce gas and bloating. Chew caraway seeds or brew caraway tea and consume it.

It is important to consult with a healthcare professional if you experience chronic or severe bloating and gas, as these symptoms can indicate underlying digestive conditions. Natural remedies should be used as supportive measures alongside dietary and lifestyle changes. Additionally, individual responses to these remedies may vary, so finding the one that works best for you is important.

Bronchitis

Bronchitis is an inflammatory condition that affects the bronchial tubes in the lungs. It can be acute or chronic, characterized by coughing, mucus production, chest discomfort, and difficulty breathing. Viral infections often cause acute bronchitis, while chronic bronchitis is a form of chronic obstructive pulmonary disease (COPD) typically associated with smoking. Here are some items that may help manage bronchitis:

Eucalyptus (Eucalyptus globulus): Eucalyptus can be used for steam inhalation to relieve chest congestion and promote easier breathing. Add a few drops of eucalyptus oil to hot water and inhale the steam. Be cautious not to touch the hot water or the container.

Peppermint (Mentha × piperita): Peppermint tea or oil can help relax the airways, ease coughing, and reduce chest discomfort. Inhale peppermint oil or drink peppermint tea.

Thyme (Thymus vulgaris): Thyme tea or oil has antimicrobial and anti-inflammatory properties and can help with respiratory symptoms. Consume thyme tea or inhale thyme oil vapor.

Ginger (Zingiber officinale): Ginger is known for its anti-inflammatory and soothing effects on the respiratory system. Consume ginger tea or use it as an ingredient in cooking.

Honey: Honey can be added to warm tea or consumed to soothe a sore throat and coughing associated with bronchitis. Take a teaspoon of honey as needed.

Licorice Root (Glycyrrhiza glabra): Licorice Root has anti-inflammatory properties and can help relieve bronchitis symptoms. Brew licorice root tea and consume it.

Mullein (Verbascum thapsus): Mullein is traditionally used to ease respiratory issues and can help alleviate bronchitis symptoms.
Brew mullein tea and consume it.

It is important to consult with a healthcare professional if you suspect you have bronchitis or are experiencing severe symptoms. A range of factors can cause bronchitis, and the treatment may vary. Natural remedies should be used as complementary measures and should not replace prescribed medications or professional guidance. When using natural remedies, you must monitor your symptoms and seek medical attention if they worsen or persist.

Candidiasis

Candidiasis is a fungal infection that occurs due to the overgrowth of Candida yeast, primarily Candida albicans, in the body. This yeast normally exists in small quantities in the human body, especially in the mouth, throat, gut, and genital area. However, an overgrowth leads to candidiasis, manifesting in various forms, including.

Oral Candidiasis (Thrush). This infection affects the mouth and throat, often appearing as white, creamy, raised lesions on the tongue, inner cheeks, and back of the throat.

Vaginal Candidiasis: Often called a yeast infection, it affects the vaginal area, causing itching, burning, and abnormal vaginal discharge.

Cutaneous Candidiasis: This form affects the skin, particularly in warm, moist areas, and results in red, itchy, and sometimes pustular rashes.

Systemic Candidiasis: This more severe form occurs in individuals with weakened immune systems, potentially affecting the bloodstream and multiple organs.

Here are a few natural remedies to benefit individuals with candidiasis:

Garlic (Allium sativum): Garlic possesses natural antifungal properties. Consuming fresh garlic cloves daily supports the body's defenses against Candida overgrowth. It is also available as a supplement, with the recommended dosage provided on the product label.

Oregano Oil (Origanum vulgare): Oregano oil, containing carvacrol and thymol, offers antifungal properties. After a patch test, it works topically when diluted with carrier oil and applied to affected areas like the skin or nails after a patch test. Oregano oil is also consumable orally, but it needs dilution according to the recommended dosage on the product label.

Grapefruit Seed Extract (Citrus paradisi): Grapefruit seed extract exhibits antimicrobial properties. It is dilutable with water as mouthwash or vaginal douche in oral or vaginal candidiasis cases. The recommended dosage is on the product label.

Caprylic Acid: Caprylic acid, present in coconut oil, helps inhibit the growth of Candida when included in the diet. Caprylic acid supplements are also an option, following the recommended dosage on the product label.

Berberine: Berberine, a compound in plants like goldenseal, is available as a supplement with varying dosages. Consulting a healthcare provider for usage guidance is advisable.

Consulting with a healthcare professional is crucial if you suspect candidiasis or experience symptoms. Candidiasis manifests in diverse ways and might need specific medical treatment. Natural remedies should serve as complementary measures and not replace prescribed antifungal medications. Responses to these remedies can differ, so monitoring symptoms and seeking professional guidance when necessary is essential.

Canker Sores

Canker sores, also known as aphthous ulcers, are small, painful sores or lesions that develop on the soft tissues inside the mouth, such as the gums, tongue, lips, and the lining of the cheeks. They differ from cold sores, which appear on the lips and are caused by the herpes simplex virus. Canker sores are not contagious.

The exact cause of canker sores remains unclear, but several factors can trigger them, including minor trauma, food sensitivities, stress, and hormonal changes. Canker sores typically heal on their own within one to two weeks.

Some natural remedies and treatments can help alleviate pain and promote healing. These approaches should be used as complementary measures and discussed with a healthcare provider. Here are some natural remedies being explored for their potential benefit in managing canker sores:

Saltwater Rinse: Rinsing with a warm saltwater solution can help reduce pain and inflammation. Dissolving half a teaspoon of salt in 8 ounces of warm water and using it as a mouth rinse may provide relief.

Baking Soda Paste: Creating a paste by mixing baking soda with a small amount of water and then applying it directly to the canker sore can help reduce irritation.

Turmeric (Curcuma longa): Honey and Turmeric Paste: Some people use a mixture of honey and turmeric to soothe canker sores. Applying a small amount of this paste to the sore may be beneficial.

It is essential to consult with a healthcare provider or dentist if you experience recurrent or unusually large canker sores, as they might be a sign of an underlying health condition. In severe or recurring cases, a healthcare provider might prescribe oral medications, such as corticosteroids or antimicrobial rinses. Home remedies and natural treatments should be used under professional guidance and complement, not replace, prescribed treatments for canker sores.

Cardiovascular health

Cardiovascular health refers to the well-being and optimal functioning of the cardiovascular system, which includes the heart and blood vessels. A healthy cardiovascular system is essential for circulating blood, oxygen, and nutrients throughout the body. Cardiovascular health is a key component of overall well-being and is associated with a reduced risk of heart disease, stroke, and other cardiovascular conditions.

Diet: Eating a balanced, heart-healthy diet is crucial. It should be low in saturated and trans fats, cholesterol, sodium, and processed foods and include a variety of fruits, vegetables, whole grains, lean proteins, and healthy fats like those found in olive oil, nuts, and fish.

Physical Activity: Regular exercise is essential for cardiovascular health. It helps strengthen the heart, improve circulation, and maintain a healthy weight. You should aim for at least 150 minutes of moderate-intensity aerobic activity or 75 minutes of vigorous-intensity aerobic activity per week, along with muscle-strengthening activities.

Blood Pressure Management: Monitoring and controlling blood pressure within a healthy range is vital. High blood pressure is a significant risk factor for heart disease.

Cholesterol Management: Maintaining healthy cholesterol levels is important, focusing on reducing LDL (bad) cholesterol and increasing HDL (good) cholesterol.

Blood Sugar Control: Managing blood sugar levels is crucial, as uncontrolled diabetes can increase the risk of heart disease.

Maintaining a Healthy Weight: Achieving and maintaining a healthy body weight through diet and exercise is beneficial.

Stress Management: Reducing chronic stress through relaxation techniques, exercise, and mindfulness can improve cardiovascular health.

A heart-healthy lifestyle, including the factors mentioned above, is essential. However, some natural substances and dietary considerations are being studied for their potential benefits in supporting cardiovascular health. These approaches should be discussed with a healthcare provider and used as complementary measures:

Garlic (Allium sativum): Garlic might help lower blood pressure and reduce cholesterol levels. It can be consumed in food or supplement form.

Omega-3 Fatty Acids: Fatty fish, such as salmon and mackerel, are rich in omega-3 fatty acids, which have been linked to heart health. Omega-3 supplements are also available.

Hawthorn (Crataegus): Hawthorn supplements are used in traditional medicine to support heart health, but their use should be discussed with a healthcare provider.

Oats (Avena sativa): Oats are a source of soluble fiber that can help lower cholesterol levels. They can be consumed as oatmeal or in various dishes.

A healthcare provider can help you develop a personalized plan for maintaining and improving cardiovascular health based on your specific risk factors and medical history.

Cold Sores (Herpes Simplex Virus)

Cold sores, also known as fever blisters, are small, painful, fluid-filled blisters that typically appear on or around the lips. They result from the herpes simplex virus (HSV), specifically the herpes simplex virus type 1 (HSV-1). HSV-1 is highly contagious and transmits through close personal contact, such as kissing or sharing utensils. Once infected with HSV-1, the virus remains dormant in the body and reactivates, forming cold sores during stress, illness, or sun exposure.

There is no cure for the herpes simplex virus, so the treatment of cold sores focuses on managing and alleviating the symptoms.

Avoiding Triggers: Identifying and avoiding triggers that may prompt cold sore outbreaks, such as stress, excessive sunlight, or illness, helps reduce the frequency of outbreaks.

Some natural remedies and complementary measures can help manage symptoms or promote healing. These approaches should be used with antiviral medications and treatments prescribed by a healthcare provider:

Aloe Vera (Aloe barbadensis miller): Applying aloe vera gel to the cold sore helps soothe and moisturize the affected area.

Lemon Balm (Melissa officinalis): Lemon balm cream or ointment, applied topically, is studied for its potential to reduce cold sore symptoms and healing time.

Tea Tree Oil (Melaleuca alternifolia): Tea tree oil, known for its antiviral properties, can be diluted, and applied topically to cold sores. It should be used with caution, as it can irritate some individuals.

It is important to consult a healthcare provider for an accurate diagnosis and determine the most appropriate treatment for cold sores. Antiviral medications are the most effective way to manage and reduce the duration of cold sore outbreaks. Natural remedies should serve as complementary measures and not replace prescribed cold sore medications.

Constipation

Constipation is a common digestive issue characterized by infrequent bowel movements, difficulty passing stools, or the feeling of incomplete evacuation. It leads to discomfort, abdominal pain, and other digestive problems. Normal bowel habits vary among individuals, but having fewer than three bowel movements per week is often considered a sign of constipation.

There are numerous potential causes of constipation, including

Diet: A diet low in fiber and inadequate fluid intake contribute to constipation. A lack of dietary fiber makes stools hard and difficult to pass.

Physical Activity: A sedentary lifestyle slows the digestive system and contributes to constipation.

Medications:
Some medications, including certain pain relievers, antacids, and antidepressants, can cause constipation as a side effect.

Medical Conditions: Certain conditions, such as irritable bowel syndrome (IBS), hypothyroidism, or pelvic floor dysfunction, lead to chronic constipation.

The treatment and management of constipation typically involve lifestyle and dietary changes, including

Dietary Fiber: Increasing fiber intake through fruits, vegetables, whole grains, and legumes helps soften stools and promote regular bowel movements.

Hydration: Drinking plenty of water is essential for preventing dehydration and maintaining bowel regularity.

Physical Activity: Regular exercise helps stimulate bowel movements and promote overall digestive health.

Some natural remedies and dietary considerations may help alleviate symptoms and support regular bowel movements. These approaches should be used as complementary measures and discussed with a healthcare provider:

Psyllium Husk: Psyllium is a natural fiber supplement mixed with water to help soften stools and promote regularity.

Aloe Vera (Aloe barbadensis miller): Aloe vera juice or supplements traditionally support digestive health.

Senna: Senna is an herbal laxative found in some over-the-counter products. It should be used under the guidance of a healthcare provider.

Prunes and Prune Juice: Prunes contain natural laxative compounds and consuming them, or prune juice helps alleviate constipation.

Cough and Cold

Cough and cold are common respiratory conditions caused by viral infections, such as the common cold or influenza. They are characterized by a runny or stuffy nose, sneezing, coughing, sore throat, and sometimes a low-grade fever. Cough and cold symptoms often result from the body's immune response to the virus and typically resolve independently within a week or two.

Several natural remedies help manage symptoms and promote recovery. These approaches should be used as complementary measures and discussed with a healthcare provider:

Echinacea (Echinacea purpurea): Echinacea is an herb believed to stimulate the immune system and reduce the severity and duration of cold symptoms. It is available in various forms, including capsules, tablets, liquid extracts, and teas. The application typically involves Echinacea capsules or tablets Following the dosage instructions on the product label. Echinacea tea: Steeping a tea bag or loose echinacea herb in hot water and drink it several times daily.

Thyme (Thymus vulgaris): Thyme is an herb known for its antimicrobial properties and potential to soothe coughs. It can be used as tea or inhaled as steam. Here is how to apply it: Thyme tea: Steeping fresh or dried thyme leaves in hot water and drinking the tea helps soothe a sore throat and cough. Thyme steam inhalation: Boiling water, adding fresh thyme leaves, and inhaling the steam helps relieve congestion and ease breathing.

Honey: Honey is effective in soothing a sore throat and cough. It can be taken alone or mixed with warm water or tea.

Rest and Hydration: Getting plenty of rest and staying well-hydrated are essential for supporting the immune system and easing symptoms.

Saline Nasal Irrigation: A saline nasal spray or a neti pot helps clear nasal passages, reduce congestion, and alleviate symptoms.

Steam Inhalation: Inhaling steam from a bowl of hot water helps relieve nasal congestion and ease coughing.

Gargling with Salt Water: Warm saltwater helps soothe a sore throat.

Note that the treatment of cough and cold should focus on symptom management and providing comfort. These remedies help alleviate discomfort and speed recovery but do not cure the underlying viral infection. If symptoms persist for an extended period, or if there is a concern about complications, it is advisable to consult a healthcare provider for a proper diagnosis and treatment recommendations. Sometimes, cold, and flu-like symptoms may be caused by a bacterial infection or other underlying health conditions, and specific medical treatment may be required.

Dental Health

Practices and measures help maintain healthy teeth and gums, prevent oral health issues, and support oral hygiene. Dental health is essential for preventing dental problems like tooth decay, gum disease, and other oral conditions. Supportive dental care includes daily oral hygiene routines, regular dental check-ups, and a balanced diet.

Oral Hygiene: Practicing good oral hygiene is crucial. This includes brushing your teeth at least twice daily with fluoride toothpaste, flossing daily to remove plaque and debris from between the teeth, and using an antimicrobial mouthwash if your dentist recommends it.

Diet: A diet rich in fruits, vegetables, lean proteins, and whole grains and low in sugary and acidic foods helps maintain dental health. Avoiding excessive consumption of sugary beverages and snacks is necessary.

Natural remedies, like aloe vera gel or clove oil, temporarily relieve gum pain or inflammation. However, their use should be discussed with a healthcare provider.

It is important to note that maintaining good dental health is crucial for overall well-being. Dental issues can impact oral and overall health, as poor dental health is associated with various systemic health problems. Regular dental check-ups, oral hygiene practices, and a healthy diet form the foundation of dental health, and natural remedies should be used with caution and in consultation with a healthcare provider.

Clove (Syzygium aromaticum) and Myrrh (Commiphora myrrha) are two natural substances traditionally used and, in some cases, scientifically supported for oral health. Here is how they are applied: Clove (Syzygium aromaticum) is known for its antimicrobial and analgesic (pain-relieving) properties, making it a useful natural remedy for various dental issues. Toothache Relief: Clove oil, usually diluted with a carrier oil, is applied topically to a sore tooth or gums for temporary relief. You can also use a small piece of a whole clove and place it on the affected area. Mouthwash: Clove is used in homemade mouthwash. You steep cloves in hot water, let it cool and use the liquid as a mouthwash for its antimicrobial properties. Toothpaste: Some natural toothpaste products contain clove for its potential oral health benefits.

Myrrh (Commiphora myrrha): Myrrh is used traditionally for its potential antimicrobial and anti-inflammatory properties, making it a choice for dental health. Mouthwash: Myrrh resin is used to prepare myrrh mouthwash. It may help reduce inflammation and support oral health. To make a myrrh mouthwash, add myrrh resin to hot water, let it steep cool, and use the liquid as a mouthwash. Gum Health: Some herbal toothpaste and oral care products contain myrrh for its potential benefits in supporting gum health.

While these natural remedies may offer some relief for oral health issues, it is important to note that they should be used with caution and in consultation with a healthcare provider. Serious dental issues require professional evaluation and treatment by a dentist. Additionally, overuse or misuse of these substances can lead to adverse effects, so following recommended dosages and application guidelines is crucial.

Maintaining good oral hygiene practices, such as regular brushing and flossing, professional dental check-ups, and cleanings, remains the foundation of dental health. Natural remedies should complement, not replace, these essential practices.

Depression

Depression is a mental health condition characterized by persistent feelings of sadness, hopelessness, and a lack of interest or pleasure in daily activities. It leads to a range of emotional and physical problems and impacts a person's ability to function in daily life. Depression is a complex condition with various causes, including genetic, biological, environmental, and psychological factors.

If you or someone you know experiences symptoms of depression, it is crucial to consult with a healthcare provider for a proper diagnosis and to discuss appropriate treatment options.

St. John's Wort (Hypericum perforatum): St. John's Wort is an herb studied for its potential to manage mild to moderate depression. It is available as a dietary supplement. However, its use can interact with certain medications, and it should be used under the guidance of a healthcare professional.

Lion's Mane Mushroom (Hericium erinaceus): The Lion's Mane mushroom is being explored for its potential cognitive and mood benefits, but more research is needed.

Rhodiola (Rhodiola rosea): Rhodiola is an herb that some people use to manage stress and improve mood. It is available as a dietary supplement.

Kava (Piper methysticum): Kava is a plant used traditionally in some cultures to promote relaxation and reduce anxiety. It is available as a dietary supplement. However, its use is associated with potential liver toxicity.

The most effective treatments for depression typically involve a combination of psychotherapy, such as cognitive-behavioral therapy or interpersonal therapy, and medication, if necessary. Lifestyle changes, regular exercise, and a supportive social network are also beneficial in managing depression. Always consult a qualified healthcare professional for a comprehensive evaluation and treatment plan if you or someone you know experiences depression.

Diabetes Management

Diabetes management refers to the strategies and techniques used to control blood glucose (sugar) levels and minimize the complications associated with diabetes. Diabetes is a chronic medical condition characterized by the body's inability to regulate blood sugar due to insufficient insulin production properly (Type 1 diabetes) or insulin resistance (Type 2 diabetes).

Effective diabetes management typically involves

Diet and Nutrition: Monitoring carbohydrate intake, eating a balanced diet, and managing portion sizes to control blood sugar levels.

Physical Activity: Regular physical activity can help improve insulin sensitivity and maintain a healthy weight.

Medications and Insulin: In some cases, diabetes medications or insulin therapy may be necessary to manage blood sugar levels.

Stress Management: Reducing stress through relaxation techniques and coping strategies can help stabilize blood sugar levels.

Bitter Melon (Momordica charantia) Bitter Melon can be used in various forms, such as cooking it in dishes, juicing it, or making teas. Bitter melon can be sliced and included in stir-fries, curries, or soups.

Bitter melon can be juiced and consumed, with other fruits or vegetables, to improve the taste. You can make bitter melon tea by steeping sliced bitter melon in hot water.

Gymnema (Gymnema sylvestre): Gymnema is often available as dietary supplements, teas, or tinctures.

Cinnamon (Cinnamomum spp.): Cinnamon can be added to various foods and beverages, such as oatmeal, yogurt, tea, or smoothies. Cinnamon sticks can be steeped in hot water to make cinnamon tea.

Maitake Mushroom (Grifola frondosa) extracts are typically available in supplement form. Maitake MushroomFollow the recommended dosage on the product label.

Ginseng (Panax quinquefolius): American Ginseng is available as dietary supplements or in whole root form.

Mulberry (Morus spp.): Mulberry leaves and extracts are available in supplement form. Follow the recommended dosage on the product label.

It is important to emphasize that while these natural substances have shown promise in some studies, their use should be discussed with a healthcare provider and complement, not replace, conventional medical treatment for diabetes. Dosages and potential interactions with medications need to be considered.

Diarrhea

Diarrhea is a common digestive issue with frequent, loose, and watery bowel movements. Abdominal cramps often accompany it and can be caused by several factors, including infections, dietary issues, medications, and underlying medical conditions. In many cases, diarrhea is acute and resolves independently, but chronic diarrhea can be a symptom of a more serious condition and may require medical attention.

Stay Hydrated: Drink clear fluids like water, clear broths, or oral rehydration solutions to prevent dehydration caused by diarrhea.

Dietary Changes: Avoid or limit foods and beverages that can exacerbate diarrhea, such as caffeine, alcohol, greasy or spicy foods, and dairy products (especially if lactose intolerant).

Herbal Tea: Some medicinal herbs like chamomile, ginger, and peppermint may help soothe the digestive tract. They can be consumed as herbal teas.

Probiotics: Probiotics in foods like yogurt and dietary supplements may help restore the balance of beneficial gut bacteria.

BRAT Diet: The BRAT diet includes bananas, rice, applesauce, and toast, land, easy-to-digest foods that may be helpful during and after a bout of diarrhea.

Blackberry (Rubus spp.): Blackberries are known for their high antioxidant content and are a useful source of dietary fiber, vitamins, and minerals.

The tannins in blackberries may help reduce inflammation and promote digestive health. Consuming blackberries and their high fiber content may help support overall digestive health.

It is important to note that the effectiveness of these natural remedies can vary from person to person and should be complementary to other recommended treatments. If you experience severe or persistent diarrhea or have other concerning symptoms, it is crucial to consult with a medical professional for diagnosis and treatment.

Additionally, if you are considering using herbal remedies or dietary changes to manage diarrhea, consult a healthcare provider or herbalist to ensure it is appropriate for your situation. Natural remedies should be considered along with traditional medical care for chronic or severe diarrhea cases.

Digestive Issues

Digestive issues encompass a broad range of conditions, from indigestion and bloating to gas and gastrointestinal discomfort. While there is no one-size-fits-all-natural remedy for digestive issues, several medicinal plants, herbs, and dietary adjustments can help alleviate discomfort and support digestive health.

Ginger (Zingiber officinale): Preparation: Fresh ginger root is known for its digestive benefits and can be used to make ginger tea or added to dishes. Ginger Tea: To make ginger tea, peel and thinly slice fresh ginger (about one teaspoon per cup) and steep it in hot water for about 5-10 minutes. You can add honey or lemon for flavor.

Peppermint (Mentha piperita): Peppermint leaves are used to make herbal tea, which may help alleviate symptoms of indigestion. Use dried peppermint leaves (about one teaspoon per cup) to make peppermint tea. Steep for 5-10 minutes and enjoy.

Fennel (Foeniculum vulgare): Fennel seeds can be chewed or brewed into tea to reduce bloating and support digestion. Crush a teaspoon of fennel seeds and steep them in hot water for 5-10 minutes.

Papaya (Carica papaya): Papaya contains digestive enzymes (papain) that can aid digestion. You can eat ripe papaya fruit or drink papaya enzyme supplements.

Probiotics: Probiotic-rich foods like yogurt and fermented foods (e.g., sauerkraut, kimchi) can help maintain a healthy gut microbiome and promote digestion.

Dietary Adjustments: Consider dietary changes such as avoiding trigger foods, chewing food slowly, and eating smaller, more frequent meals to aid digestion.

Peppermint Oil (Mentha × piperita): Peppermint oil capsules or enteric-coated tablets may be used to alleviate symptoms of irritable bowel syndrome (IBS) and other digestive issues. Follow the recommended dosage on the product label.

Chamomile (Matricaria chamomilla): Chamomile tea is known for its potential to relax the gastrointestinal tract and reduce digestive discomfort. Chamomile Tea: Steep dried chamomile flowers (about one teaspoon per cup) in hot water for 5-10 minutes.

As with any natural remedy, using them safely and in moderation is important. If you have any underlying medical conditions or are taking medications, consult a healthcare provider or herbalist to ensure these remedies are appropriate.

Ear Infections

Ear infections can be painful and uncomfortable, often affecting children but also occurring in adults. While there is not a single natural remedy that can replace medical treatment, some approaches may help alleviate symptoms or support overall ear health:

Garlic (Allium sativum): Garlic is known for its natural antimicrobial properties. Garlic oil can be used in some cases to help combat ear infections. Crush a fresh garlic clove, mix it with carrier oil (like olive oil), and warm it slightly. Place a few drops in the affected ear after it has cooled to body temperature. Do not insert it too deeply; consult a healthcare provider before using this remedy.

Mullein (Verbascum thapsus): Mullein oil is traditionally used for its potential soothing and anti-inflammatory properties and may help relieve ear discomfort.

Preparation: Warm mullein oil and put a few drops into the affected ear. Allow it to sit for a few minutes, then drain it.

Tea Tree Oil (Melaleuca alternifolia): Tea tree oil has natural antimicrobial properties and can be used as a potential ear cleaner.
Preparation: Mix a few drops of tea tree oil with carrier oil, apply a small amount to a cotton ball, and gently clean the external ear. Do not insert it into the ear canal.

Warm Compress: Applying a warm, moist compress to the affected ear may help alleviate pain and discomfort associated with ear infections. Ensure it is not too hot to avoid burns.

Hydration and Nutrition: Staying well-hydrated and maintaining a balanced diet can support overall immune health, potentially reducing the risk of ear infections.

Probiotics: Probiotic supplements and foods can help maintain a healthy balance of gut bacteria, which may indirectly support the immune system and ear health.

Keep Ears Dry: Preventing water from entering the ear, especially during swimming, can help reduce the risk of moisture-related ear infections.

If you suspect an ear infection, it is essential to consult with a healthcare provider for a proper diagnosis and treatment plan. Natural remedies should not replace medical care, especially in severe or persistent infections.

These natural remedies may relieve mild ear discomfort or support overall ear health, but they should not be used as a substitute for medical treatment. It is crucial to consult a healthcare provider in ear infections, especially when symptoms are severe or prolonged. They can determine the appropriate action, including antibiotics or other medical interventions.

Eczema

Eczema, also known as atopic dermatitis, is a chronic skin condition characterized by red, itchy, and inflamed skin. While eczema has no cure, various natural and supportive measures can help manage and alleviate its symptoms. Here are some approaches:

Coconut Oil (Cocos nucifera): Coconut oil is a natural emollient that can help moisturize the skin and reduce dryness, which is common in eczema. Apply virgin coconut oil to the affected areas of the skin. Ensure your skin is clean, and gently massage the oil in. Use it as needed for moisturizing.

Oatmeal Baths: Oatmeal can help soothe and relieve itchy skin. Oatmeal baths can be particularly calming for eczema. Preparation: Grind plain, unflavored oatmeal into a fine powder. Add it to a warm bath and soak for 15-20 minutes. Pat your skin dry afterward.

Chamomile (Matricaria chamomilla): Chamomile has anti-inflammatory and soothing properties that can help reduce skin irritation. Brew chamomile tea, allow it to cool, and use a soft cloth to apply it to the affected areas as a compress.

Aloe Vera (Aloe barbadensis miller): Aloe vera has moisturizing and anti-inflammatory properties, making it helpful for reducing skin irritation. Apply pure aloe vera gel to the affected skin. Ensure the gel you use is free of added chemicals or fragrances.

Avoid Triggers: Identify and avoid triggers that worsen your eczema. Common triggers include harsh soaps, allergens, stress, and certain foods.

Cotton Clothing: Wear loose-fitting cotton clothing to reduce skin irritation and allow the skin to breathe.

Honey: Raw honey has natural antibacterial and moisturizing properties and can be applied to eczema-prone areas.

Preparation: Apply a thin layer of raw honey to the affected skin, leave it on for about 20-30 minutes, and then rinse it with lukewarm water.

Dietary Adjustments: Some people with eczema find that certain foods can trigger or exacerbate symptoms. Identifying and eliminating trigger foods may help manage eczema.

Stay Hydrated: Drinking plenty of water helps keep the skin hydrated from the inside out. It is important to note that individual responses to these natural remedies may vary. If you have severe or persistent eczema, or if your symptoms worsen, it is essential to consult with a healthcare provider or a dermatologist for a proper diagnosis and treatment plan. Medical treatments, including prescription creams and medications, may be necessary to manage eczema effectively. Natural remedies can complement medical care but should not replace it, especially in severe cases.

Fertility Issues

Fertility issues can be challenging, and while there is no single natural remedy that can guarantee success, there are supportive measures and lifestyle changes that may help improve fertility. These measures do not replace medical evaluation and treatment but can complement medical care. Here are some approaches that may support fertility:

Diet and Nutrition: Maintaining a healthy diet is essential. Include a variety of fruits, vegetables, whole grains, lean proteins, and healthy fats in your diet. Pay attention to your nutrient intake, particularly folic acid, iron, and other essential vitamins and minerals. Consider consulting with a registered dietitian or nutritionist for personalized guidance.

Weight Management: Achieving and maintaining a healthy body weight is crucial for fertility. Both being underweight and overweight can negatively impact fertility. Consult with a healthcare provider to determine your ideal weight and seek guidance on weight management.

Regular Exercise: Physical activity can help manage weight and improve overall health. Aim for moderate exercise, but avoid excessive, high-intensity exercise that may disrupt the menstrual cycle. Consult with a healthcare provider for an exercise plan that suits your needs.

Stress Management: Elevated levels of stress can affect fertility. Explore stress reduction techniques such as yoga, meditation, deep breathing exercises, and counseling. Counseling or therapy can help address emotional factors that may be impacting fertility.

Sleep Hygiene: Prioritize quality sleep. Aim for 7-9 hours of uninterrupted sleep per night to support hormonal balance.

Maca (Lepidium meyenii): Maca is a root vegetable native to the Andes in Peru. It is known for its potential benefits in supporting hormonal balance and overall reproductive health.

Preparation: Maca is available in various forms, including capsules, powders, and as a raw vegetable. It can be incorporated into
smoothies, taken as a dietary supplement, or consumed as a food. Follow the dosage instructions on the product label. It is often taken daily, but individual responses may vary.

Red Raspberry Leaf (Rubus idaeus): Red raspberry leaf is known for its potential benefits in toning the uterus and supporting the female reproductive system. It is commonly used as a herbal tea.

Preparation: To make red raspberry leaf tea, use dried red raspberry leaves. Steep one to two teaspoons of dried leaves in hot water for about 5-10 minutes. Drink it daily during your menstrual cycle until ovulation.

Limit Alcohol and Caffeine: Excessive alcohol and caffeine consumption can negatively impact fertility. Consider reducing or eliminating these from your diet.

Avoid Smoking and Recreational Drugs: Smoking and recreational drug use can significantly impair fertility. Seek support to quit these habits.

If you have been trying to conceive for an extended period without success, consult a healthcare provider. They can evaluate your reproductive health, identify any underlying issues, and provide guidance on fertility treatments if needed.

Remember that fertility issues can be complex, and a multifaceted approach is often necessary. It is important to consult with a healthcare provider for personalized advice and a comprehensive evaluation of your fertility. Natural remedies and lifestyle changes can support your efforts to improve fertility but should be used with medical care, especially if fertility issues persist.

Fibromyalgia

Fibromyalgia is a chronic pain disorder characterized by widespread musculoskeletal pain, fatigue, and tenderness in specific body areas. It is a complex condition with no known cure, and its exact cause is poorly understood. Treatment typically focuses on managing symptoms and improving quality of life.
Some natural and supportive approaches can help manage its symptoms. Here are some commonly used measures:

Exercise: Low-impact exercises such as walking, swimming, and tai chi can help improve muscle strength and flexibility. Regular exercise is known to reduce pain and fatigue in fibromyalgia.

Diet and Nutrition: A balanced diet rich in fruits, vegetables, whole grains, and lean proteins can support overall health. Some individuals with fibromyalgia find relief by reducing their consumption of processed foods, sugar, and caffeine.

Stress Management: Stress-reduction techniques such as meditation, yoga, deep breathing exercises, and mindfulness can help alleviate stress and improve overall well-being.

Adequate Sleep: Maintaining a regular sleep schedule and creating a comfortable sleeping environment can improve sleep quality, essential for managing fibromyalgia.

Heat and Cold Therapy: Warm baths or heating pads can relax muscles and reduce pain, while cold packs can help reduce inflammation and numb painful areas.

Massage and Bodywork: Massage therapy and other bodywork techniques can reduce muscle tension and improve circulation, potentially alleviating pain.

Acupuncture: Some individuals with fibromyalgia find relief from pain and improved energy levels through acupuncture, a traditional Chinese medicine practice involving the insertion of thin needles into specific points on the body.

Supplements: Some people with fibromyalgia may benefit from supplements like magnesium, vitamin D, and omega-3 fatty acids. Consult a healthcare provider before using supplements to determine the most appropriate options for your situation.

Support Groups: Joining a support group or seeking therapy can provide emotional support and coping strategies for individuals with fibromyalgia.

Turmeric (Curcuma longa): Turmeric is a spice derived from the root of the Curcuma longa plant and contains an active compound called curcumin. It is well-known for its anti-inflammatory and antioxidant properties. While turmeric has not been proven to cure fibromyalgia, it may help alleviate some of its symptoms, such as pain and inflammation.

Turmeric can be added to your diet as a spice, dietary supplement, or capsules. The key component, curcumin, is not well-absorbed by the body, so it is often combined with black pepper or piperine to enhance absorption.

St. John's Wort (Hypericum perforatum): St. John's Wort is an herbal remedy traditionally used for its potential mood-enhancing and antidepressant effects. While it is not a direct treatment for fibromyalgia, it may help with the emotional aspects of the condition, such as depression and anxiety, which can often accompany fibromyalgia. St. John's Wort is available in various forms, including capsules, tablets, and liquid extracts. It is essential to consult with a healthcare provider before using St. John's Wort, as it can interact with certain medications and have side effects.

It is important to work closely with a healthcare provider to develop a personalized treatment plan for fibromyalgia. Natural and supportive measures can complement medical care but should not replace it, especially in cases of severe or persistent symptoms. Fibromyalgia is a complex condition, and its management often requires a combination of strategies to improve the quality of life and reduce pain.

Fungal Infections

Fungal infections can affect various body parts, including the skin, nails, mouth, and genital area. They are typically caused by fungi such as Candida and dermatophytes. While antifungal medications prescribed by a healthcare provider are the primary treatment for fungal infections, several supportive measures and natural remedies can help manage these infections. These approaches should be used with medical care. Here are some supportive strategies:

Tea Tree Oil (Melaleuca alternifolia): Tea tree oil has natural antifungal properties and can be diluted with a carrier oil and applied to fungal skin infections like athlete's foot or toenail fungus.

Probiotics: Probiotics, particularly those containing Lactobacillus and Bifidobacterium strains, can help restore the balance of beneficial bacteria in the gut and may indirectly support the immune system's ability to fight fungal infections.

Dietary Changes: Reducing the consumption of sugary and processed foods can help create an environment less conducive to fungal growth. A diet rich in probiotic foods like yogurt and kefir may also support gut health.

Hygiene Practices: Keeping the affected area clean and dry is essential. Use gentle, non-irritating soaps and avoid overly hot showers, which can exacerbate skin irritation.

Garlic (Allium sativum): Garlic contains natural antifungal properties and can be included in your diet. Some individuals also use garlic topically on fungal skin infections.

Oregano Oil (Origanum vulgare): Oregano oil has antifungal properties and can be diluted with carrier oil and applied to fungal skin infections.

Apple Cider Vinegar: Some people use a diluted solution of apple cider vinegar to rinse or soak affected areas for nail and skin fungal infections.

Wearing Breathable Fabrics: For skin fungal infections, wearing breathable fabrics like cotton can help reduce moisture and prevent fungal growth.

Gastroesophageal Reflux Disease (GERD)

Gastroesophageal Reflux Disease (GERD) is a chronic condition where stomach acid flows back into the esophagus, leading to symptoms like heartburn, regurgitation, and irritation of the esophagus. While medications and lifestyle changes are the primary treatments for GERD, there are supportive measures and natural remedies that can help manage symptoms. These approaches should be used with medical care. Here are some supportive strategies for GERD:

Dietary Modifications: Avoid trigger foods and beverages, such as spicy foods, citrus, coffee, and carbonated drinks. Monitor your diet and make a list of items that worsen your symptoms. Reducing or eliminating these trigger foods can help reduce acid reflux.

Ginger (Zingiber officinale): You can consume ginger as tea or incorporate it into your meals. Make tea with fresh ginger slices in hot water, steeping for several minutes. Drink ginger tea after meals or when you experience heartburn symptoms. You can also add small amounts of fresh ginger to your dishes.

Chewing Gum: Chew sugar-free gum after meals to stimulate saliva production. Chewing gum for about 30 minutes after eating can help neutralize stomach acid and reduce the risk of acid reflux.

Aloe Vera (Aloe barbadensis miller): Choose aloe vera juice that is specifically prepared for internal use. Follow the recommended dosage on the product label. Consume a small amount of aloe vera juice as directed. It may have soothing properties for the esophagus.

Baking Soda: Dissolve a teaspoon of baking soda in a glass of water. Sometimes, a solution of baking soda and water can temporarily relieve heartburn by neutralizing stomach acid. Use this sparingly and under the guidance of a healthcare provider.

Elevating the Head of the Bed: Place blocks or bed risers under the head of your bed to raise it by a few inches. Elevate the head of your bed to keep your upper body elevated during sleep, reducing the likelihood of nighttime acid reflux.

Smaller, More Frequent Meals: Instead of large, heavy meals, opt for smaller, more frequent meals throughout the day. This can help prevent overeating and reduce pressure on the lower esophageal sphincter.

Avoid Tight Clothing: Wear loose-fitting clothing to reduce pressure on the abdomen and lower esophagus.

Slippery Elm (Ulmus rubra): Slippery elm can be consumed as a tea or supplement. If used as a tea, steep slippery elm in hot water and drink it before or after meals. It may have soothing effects on the lining of the esophagus.

It is crucial to consult with a healthcare provider for a proper diagnosis and treatment plan if you suspect you have GERD. Medications a healthcare provider prescribes are often needed to manage the condition effectively. Natural remedies can complement medical care.

Gastrointestinal Disorders

Gastrointestinal disorders encompass many conditions affecting the digestive system, including the stomach, intestines, liver, and pancreas. The management of these disorders often involves medications and medical interventions, but there are supportive measures and natural remedies that can help alleviate some symptoms and promote digestive health. These approaches should be used with medical care. Here are some supportive strategies for gastrointestinal disorders:

Dietary Modifications: Adapt your diet to your specific condition. In some cases, this may involve avoiding trigger foods or following a specific diet plan recommended by your healthcare provider.

Fiber: Incorporate fiber-rich foods such as whole grains, fruits, and vegetables into your diet. You can also take fiber supplements, but it is essential to consult a healthcare provider.

Gradually increase your fiber intake to avoid digestive discomfort. Ensure you drink plenty of water to support the effectiveness of fiber.

Probiotics: Probiotic supplements are available in various forms, such as capsules and yogurt, are available in various forms. Consult a healthcare provider to choose the right probiotic strain for your condition. Take probiotics as directed by your healthcare provider. Probiotics can help maintain a healthy balance of gut bacteria.

Peppermint (Mentha × piperita): Peppermint oil is available in enteric-coated capsules to prevent it from breaking down in the stomach. It can also be consumed as peppermint tea. Take peppermint oil capsules as directed or drink peppermint tea to potentially alleviate symptoms like irritable bowel syndrome (IBS) and indigestion.

Ginger (Zingiber officinale): Ginger can be used fresh, as a spice in your cooking, or as ginger tea. Ginger may help with symptoms like nausea and indigestion. You can consume ginger tea or incorporate ginger into your meals.

Chamomile (Matricaria chamomilla): Chamomile tea is a common way to consume chamomile. It is available in tea bags or loose-leaf form. Chamomile tea may help with digestive discomfort and relaxation. Drink chamomile tea as needed.

Slippery Elm (Ulmus rubra): Slippery elm can be consumed as a tea or supplement. It may have soothing effects on the digestive tract.

Hydration: Ensure you stay well-hydrated to support healthy digestion. Water is essential for the proper functioning of the digestive system.

Gentle Exercise: Engage in low-impact exercises like walking or yoga to help promote regular bowel movements and overall digestive health.

Gout

Gout is a type of arthritis caused by the accumulation of urate crystals in the joints, leading to pain and inflammation. While medications are often prescribed to manage gout, there are supportive measures and natural remedies that can help alleviate symptoms and reduce the risk of future gout attacks. These approaches should be used with medical care. Some supportive strategies for gout:

Dietary Modifications: Avoid or limit foods and beverages high in purines, such as organ meats, seafood, and beer. Consume a balanced diet emphasizing fruits, vegetables, and whole grains. Follow a gout-friendly diet to help reduce the risk of gout attacks. Staying well-hydrated is also essential to help flush excess uric acid from the body.

Cherry Juice or Cherries: You can consume tart cherry juice or fresh cherries. Cherry juice or cherries may help reduce the frequency and intensity of gout attacks. Consume them regularly as part of your diet. Some people take tart cherry supplements in capsule form. Consult with a healthcare provider to determine the appropriate dosage.

Turmeric (Curcuma longa): Turmeric can be used as a spice in your cooking or as a dietary supplement.

Turmeric's anti-inflammatory properties may help alleviate gout symptoms. Incorporate turmeric into your meals or consult a healthcare provider about using it as a supplement.

Baking Soda: Dissolve half a teaspoon of baking soda in a glass of water. Baking soda may help raise the urine pH, potentially making it less acidic and aiding in the excretion of uric acid. Use this sparingly and under the guidance of a healthcare provider.

Hydration: Stay well-hydrated by drinking plenty of water to help flush excess uric acid from the body.

Celery Seed (Apium graveolens): Celery seed extract is available as a supplement. Consult with a healthcare provider to determine the appropriate dosage.

It is essential to consult with a healthcare provider for a proper diagnosis and treatment plan for gout. Medications a healthcare provider prescribes are often necessary to manage the condition effectively. Natural remedies can complement medical care but should not replace it, especially in severe or persistent gout symptoms. The management of gout typically requires a comprehensive approach, including dietary changes and lifestyle adjustments.

Hair and Scalp Disorders

Hair and scalp disorders encompass a variety of conditions that can affect your hair's health and appearance and your scalp's condition. These conditions include dandruff, hair loss, scalp psoriasis, and more. While medical treatments are often prescribed to manage these disorders, there are supportive measures and natural remedies that can help alleviate symptoms and promote healthy hair and scalp. These approaches should be used with medical care. Here are some supportive strategies for hair and scalp disorders:

Dietary Modifications: Ensure your diet includes a variety of nutrients essential for hair health, such as vitamins A, C, and E, biotin, and omega-3 fatty acids. Incorporate foods like fish, nuts, and leafy greens into your meals. Follow a well-balanced diet to give your body the nutrients it needs to maintain healthy hair and scalp.

Scalp Massage: You can use natural oils like coconut, olive, or jojoba oil for a scalp massage. Gently massage the chosen oil into your scalp using your fingertips. Leave it on for about 30 minutes or overnight, then wash your hair with a mild shampoo. Scalp massages can help improve circulation and promote a healthy scalp.

Aloe Vera (Aloe barbadensis miller): Apply a small amount of aloe vera gel directly to your scalp and hair. Leave it on for about 30 minutes, then wash your hair. Aloe vera gel may help soothe an itchy or irritated scalp and promote hair health.

Tea Tree Oil (Melaleuca alternifolia): Dilute tea tree oil with a carrier oil (such as coconut oil) and apply it to your scalp. Leave it on for 15-20 minutes, then wash your hair. Tea tree oil may have antimicrobial properties that can help with dandruff and an itchy scalp.

Lavender (Lavandula spp.) Oil: Mix a few drops of lavender oil with a carrier oil and massage it into your scalp. Leave it on for about 30 minutes, then wash your hair. Lavender oil may help with dandruff and provide a calming, pleasant scent.

Dandruff Shampoo: Use over-the-counter dandruff shampoos as directed to help manage dandruff and maintain a healthy scalp.

Hair Care Practices: Be gentle with your hair, avoid excessive heat styling, and use mild hair care products to prevent damage and maintain hair health.

Stay Hydrated: Drink adequate water to keep your body and scalp hydrated.

Consult a Dermatologist: If you have persistent or severe hair and scalp issues, consult a dermatologist for a proper diagnosis and treatment plan.

Managing these disorders requires a comprehensive approach, including dietary changes and proper hair care practices.

Hair Loss

Hair loss, or alopecia, can be a distressing condition affecting both men and women. While medical treatments and interventions are often recommended to address the underlying causes of hair loss, there are supportive measures and natural remedies that can help promote hair health and potentially reduce hair loss. These approaches should be used with medical care. Here are some supportive strategies for hair loss:

Dietary Modifications: Ensure your diet is rich in essential nutrients for hair health, including protein, vitamins (especially vitamins B), and minerals like iron and zinc. Foods like lean meats, eggs, leafy greens, and nuts can support healthy hair growth.

Scalp Massage: Gently massage your scalp with your fingertips to improve blood circulation, which may help promote hair growth. You can use natural oils like coconut, olive, or jojoba oil for scalp massages.

Aloe Vera (Aloe barbadensis miller): Apply aloe vera gel directly to your scalp and hair. Leave it on for about 30 minutes before washing your hair. Aloe vera has soothing and hydrating properties that can benefit the scalp.

Essential Oils: Essential oils like rosemary, lavender, and cedarwood oil are believed to promote hair growth. Mix a few drops of your chosen oil with a carrier oil, like jojoba or coconut oil, and massage it into your scalp. Leave it on for about 30 minutes before washing your hair.

Onion Juice: Extract the juice from onions and apply it to your scalp. Leave it on for about 30 minutes before washing your hair. Onion juice contains sulfur, which is thought to promote hair growth.

Hair Care Practices: Be gentle with your hair, avoid tight hairstyles that can stress the hair follicles, and minimize heat styling to prevent damage and hair loss.

Stay Hydrated: Drinking adequate water is essential for overall hair health and hydration.

Consult a Dermatologist: If you are experiencing severe or persistent hair loss, it is important to consult a dermatologist to identify the underlying cause.

Halitosis (Bad Breath)

Halitosis, commonly known as bad breath, can result from various causes, including poor oral hygiene, dietary habits, medical conditions, or lifestyle factors. While addressing the underlying cause is crucial, there are supportive measures and natural remedies that can help manage and improve bad breath. These approaches should be used with good oral hygiene practices and necessary medical treatments. Here are some supportive strategies for bad breath:

Oral Hygiene: Brush your teeth and tongue thoroughly at least twice daily using fluoride toothpaste. Make sure to replace your toothbrush regularly. Floss daily to remove food particles and plaque from between your teeth. Use an antimicrobial mouthwash or rinse recommended by your dentist. Some natural options include mouthwashes with ingredients like tea tree oil or activated charcoal.

Stay Hydrated: Drink adequate water throughout the day to help maintain saliva production. Saliva is essential for rinsing away bacteria and food particles that can cause bad breath.

Green Tea (Camellia sinensis): Green tea contains natural compounds that may help inhibit the growth of odor-causing bacteria. Drink a cup of unsweetened green tea daily.

Herbs and Spices: Chewing on fresh herbs like parsley, mint, or fennel seeds can help freshen your breath naturally. These herbs contain chlorophyll, which can neutralize odors.

Probiotics: Probiotic supplements or foods like yogurt with live cultures may help balance the oral microbiome and reduce bad breath.

Dietary Adjustments: Limit or avoid foods with strong odors, such as garlic, onions, and certain spices, as these can contribute to bad breath.

Consult a Dentist: If bad breath persists, consult a dentist to rule out any underlying dental issues, such as gum disease or cavities. They can provide professional cleaning and guidance for improving oral hygiene.

Consult a Healthcare Provider: If bad breath is related to an underlying medical condition, such as sinusitis or acid reflux, consult a healthcare provider for proper diagnosis and treatment.

These supportive measures and natural remedies can help manage bad breath and promote oral health. However, they should be used with good oral hygiene practices and professional dental care, especially if bad breath is persistent or associated with dental issues.

Head Lice

Head lice are small insects that infest the scalp and can cause itching and discomfort. While medical treatments are typically necessary to eliminate head lice, there are supportive measures and natural remedies that can complement treatment and help manage infestations. These approaches should be used with prescribed treatments and thorough cleaning. Here are some supportive strategies for dealing with head lice:

Comb with a Fine-Toothed Comb: After applying a lice treatment, comb your hair with a fine-toothed comb to remove lice and nits (lice eggs). This process can help remove lice that may have survived treatment.

Wet Combing: Wet your hair and use a fine-toothed comb to go through the hair section by section. This can help physically remove lice.

Natural Oils: Some natural oils, such as tea tree or neem oil, are believed to have lice-repelling properties. You can mix a few drops of these oils with a carrier oil (like coconut oil) and apply it to the scalp.

Vinegar: Vinegar can help loosen the glue lice use to attach their eggs (nits) to the hair shaft. After treatment, you can rinse the hair with a solution of vinegar and water.

Lice-Repellent Shampoo: Some shampoos contain natural ingredients like tea tree oil, neem oil, or rosemary, which may help repel lice. Consider using these shampoos regularly, especially if your community has lice outbreaks.

Washing and Cleaning: Wash and dry all bedding, clothing, and personal items (hats, hairbrushes, etc.) that may have come into contact with lice in hot water and high heat to kill lice and nits. Vacuum your home to remove any lice that may have fallen.

Prevent Reinfestation: Encourage family members to avoid head-to-head contact and sharing personal items to prevent re-infestation.

Consult a Healthcare Provider: If lice infestations persist despite treatment and supportive measures, consult a healthcare provider for additional guidance and potential prescription treatments.

Hemorrhoids

Hemorrhoids, swollen and inflamed blood vessels in the rectum or anus, can cause discomfort, itching, and pain. While medical treatments are often recommended to alleviate symptoms and promote healing, there are supportive measures and natural remedies that can help manage hemorrhoids. These approaches should be used with prescribed treatments and lifestyle changes. Here are some supportive strategies for dealing with hemorrhoids:

Dietary Modifications: Ensure your diet is fiber-rich to promote regular, soft bowel movements. Foods like whole grains, fruits, vegetables, and legumes can aid in preventing constipation, which can exacerbate hemorrhoid symptoms.

Stay Hydrated: Drinking adequate water throughout the day can help soften stool and ease bowel movements, reducing the strain on hemorrhoids.

Topical Applications: Apply a cold compress or ice pack to the affected area for short periods to reduce swelling and discomfort. Alternatively, you can use witch hazel or aloe vera gel, which can have soothing and anti-inflammatory properties.

Sitz Baths: Soaking in a warm sitz bath for 15-20 minutes can relieve hemorrhoid discomfort. You can do this in a special sitz bath basin or in your bathtub.

Witch Hazel: Apply witch hazel-soaked cotton pads or a witch hazel-based ointment to the affected area. Witch hazel is known for its anti-inflammatory and astringent properties.

Aloe Vera (Aloe barbadensis miller): Apply pure aloe vera gel to the affected area to reduce inflammation and relieve itching and pain.

Butcher's broom (Ruscus aculeatus): Butcher's Broom is an herbal remedy traditionally used for various health issues, including hemorrhoids. It contains active compounds called ruscogenins, believed to have anti-inflammatory and vasoconstrictive (blood vessel narrowing) properties that can help with hemorrhoid symptoms. You can find topical creams or ointments that contain butcher's broom extract in some health food stores or online. These products are applied directly to the affected area to help reduce swelling and discomfort. Butcher's broom is also available in oral supplements, such as capsules or tablets. These supplements are taken by mouth and may help improve blood circulation and reduce inflammation, which can benefit hemorrhoids. Some people make herbal teas using butcher's broom. While this is less common, it can be an option for those who prefer liquid forms of supplementation. Ensure you follow the recommended dosage.

Proper Hygiene: Gently clean the anal area with unscented, moist toilet wipes or a damp cloth after bowel movements. Avoid harsh or scented soaps, as they can irritate the area.

Consult a Healthcare Provider: If hemorrhoid symptoms are severe, persistent, or bleeding.

High Blood Pressure

High blood pressure, or hypertension, is a chronic condition that can increase the risk of heart disease and other health problems. While medical treatments and lifestyle changes are often prescribed to manage high blood pressure, there are supportive measures and natural remedies that can complement treatment and help maintain blood pressure within a healthy range. These approaches should be used with medical care and under a healthcare provider's guidance. Here are some supportive strategies for dealing with high blood pressure:

Dietary Modifications: Adopt a heart-healthy diet, such as the DASH (Dietary Approaches to Stop Hypertension) diet, which emphasizes fruits, vegetables, whole grains, lean proteins, and low-fat dairy products. Reducing sodium (salt) intake is crucial for managing blood pressure.

Potassium-rich foods: Consume potassium-rich foods, such as bananas, sweet potatoes, and spinach. Potassium can help balance the effects of sodium on blood pressure.

Garlic: Incorporate garlic into your diet, whether raw or as a supplement. Garlic may have mild blood pressure-lowering properties.

Hibiscus Tea: Some research suggests that hibiscus tea may help lower blood pressure. Brew it as tea and consume it regularly, but consult with your healthcare provider, especially if you are on blood pressure medications.

Beetroot Juice: Beetroot juice contains nitrates to help relax blood vessels and lower blood pressure. Consume it in moderation.

Physical Activity: Engage in regular physical activity, such as brisk walking, jogging, or cycling, as it can help lower blood pressure. Aim for at least 150 minutes of moderate-intensity exercise per week.

Weight Management: Maintain a healthy weight through a combination of a balanced diet and regular exercise.

Stress Reduction: Practice stress-reduction techniques like deep breathing, meditation, yoga, or mindfulness to help manage stress, which can impact blood pressure.

Limit Caffeine: Reduce caffeine intake if you are sensitive to its effects on blood pressure. Monitor how caffeine affects your blood pressure and adjust your consumption accordingly.

Consult a Healthcare Provider: If you have high blood pressure, it is essential to work closely with a healthcare provider to monitor your condition and develop an individualized treatment plan, which may include medications or other medical interventions.

High Cholesterol

High cholesterol, particularly elevated levels of low-density lipoprotein (LDL) cholesterol, can increase the risk of heart disease. While medications are often prescribed to manage high cholesterol, there are supportive measures and natural remedies that can complement treatment and help maintain healthy cholesterol levels. These approaches should be used under a healthcare provider's guidance and with lifestyle changes. Here are some supportive strategies for dealing with high cholesterol:

Dietary Modifications: Adopt a heart-healthy diet that includes foods low in saturated and trans fats. Emphasize foods like whole grains, fruits, vegetables, lean proteins, and sources of healthy fats, such as nuts, seeds, and fatty fish.

Soluble Fiber: Incorporate foods rich in soluble fiber into your diet, like oats, beans, lentils, and fruits. Soluble fiber can help lower LDL cholesterol levels.

Plant Sterols and Stanols: Some foods, like fortified margarine and orange juice, contain plant sterols and stanols, which can help lower LDL cholesterol when consumed regularly.

Omega-3 Fatty Acids: Consume fatty fish like salmon, mackerel, or trout, or consider fish oil supplements. Omega-3 fatty acids can have a positive impact on cholesterol levels.

Garlic: Garlic may have mild cholesterol-lowering properties. Consider adding garlic to your cooking or taking it as a supplement.

Green Tea: Drinking green tea may help reduce LDL cholesterol levels.

Red Yeast Rice: Red yeast rice is a traditional Chinese remedy that contains compounds like statin medications. Consult with a healthcare provider before using it, as it can interact with certain medications.

Regular Physical Activity: Engage in regular exercise to help improve cholesterol levels. Aim for at least 150 minutes of moderate-intensity exercise per week.

Weight Management: Maintaining a healthy weight through a balanced diet and regular physical activity.

Limit Alcohol and Caffeine: If you consume alcohol, do so in moderation. Limit caffeine intake if you are sensitive to its effects on cholesterol.

Consult a Healthcare Provider: If you have high cholesterol, work closely with a healthcare provider to monitor your condition, and develop an individualized treatment plan, which may include medications or other medical interventions.

When used with medical care and lifestyle changes, these supportive measures and natural remedies can be valuable for managing high cholesterol.

Hormone Imbalance

Hormone imbalances can lead to many symptoms and health issues. While medical treatments and hormone therapy may be necessary for addressing specific hormone imbalances, there are supportive measures and natural remedies that can help manage symptoms and promote hormone balance. These approaches should be used with medical care and under a healthcare provider's guidance. Here are some supportive strategies for dealing with hormone imbalances:

Balanced Diet: Consume a balanced diet rich in whole foods, including fruits, vegetables, whole grains, lean proteins, and healthy fats. This can help support overall health and hormone balance. Regular Physical Activity: Engage in regular exercise, such as aerobic activities, strength training, and yoga. Exercise can help regulate hormones and reduce stress.

Stress Management: Practice stress-reduction techniques like deep breathing, meditation, mindfulness, or progressive muscle relaxation to help manage stress, which can affect hormone balance.

Adequate Sleep: Prioritize sleep and aim for 7-9 hours of quality sleep per night to support hormonal health.

Chasteberry (Vitex agnus-castus): Chasteberry is often used to help regulate hormonal imbalances in women. It can benefit premenstrual syndrome (PMS) and irregular menstrual cycles. Chasteberry is available in various forms, including capsules, tinctures, and dried herbs. The appropriate dosage depends on the form but is typically taken once daily. Follow the manufacturer's instructions or consult with a healthcare provider.

Probiotics: Probiotic supplements or foods like yogurt with live cultures can help maintain a healthy balance of gut bacteria, potentially affecting hormone balance.

Limit Caffeine and Alcohol: Reduce caffeine and alcohol consumption, as excessive intake can impact hormone levels and disrupt sleep patterns.

Healthy Fats: Incorporate sources of healthy fats like avocados, nuts, and olive oil into your diet to support hormone production.

Consult a Healthcare Provider: If you suspect a hormone imbalance or are experiencing symptoms, consult a healthcare provider for proper evaluation, testing, and individualized treatment recommendations. Hormone imbalances vary widely, and treatment may require prescription medications or hormone replacement therapy.

These supportive measures and natural remedies can help manage hormone imbalances when used in conjunction with medical care and lifestyle changes. Consult your healthcare provider to determine the most appropriate and safe approach for your specific hormone imbalance.

Hyperthyroidism

Hyperthyroidism is a condition in which the thyroid gland produces excessive thyroid hormones, leading to a range of symptoms, including weight loss, anxiety, rapid heartbeat, and more. While medical treatments are often necessary to manage hyperthyroidism, there are supportive measures and natural remedies that can help alleviate symptoms and promote thyroid health.

These approaches should be used under a healthcare provider's guidance and in conjunction with medical care. Here are some supportive strategies for dealing with hyperthyroidism:

Dietary Modifications: Consume a well-balanced diet that includes foods rich in essential nutrients like iodine and selenium, which are important for thyroid health. Iodine-rich foods include seaweed, fish, and dairy, while selenium can be found in nuts, seeds, and lean meats.

Limit Stimulants: Avoid or limit stimulants like caffeine and nicotine, as they can exacerbate symptoms like rapid heart rate and anxiety.

Stress Management: Practice stress-reduction techniques like yoga, meditation, or deep breathing exercises, as stress can trigger or worsen hyperthyroid symptoms.

Lemon Balm (Melissa officinalis): Lemon balm tea or supplements may have a calming effect and help alleviate anxiety associated with hyperthyroidism.

Bugleweed (Lycopus virginicus): Bugleweed is an herb that may help reduce thyroid hormone production. It is available in tincture form.

Consult a Healthcare Provider: If you suspect or have been diagnosed with hyperthyroidism, it is crucial to work closely with a healthcare provider for proper evaluation, testing, and treatment recommendations. Hyperthyroidism often requires medications, radioactive iodine treatment, or surgery to manage thyroid function effectively.

These supportive measures and natural remedies can help manage symptoms associated with hyperthyroidism when used with medical care and treatment. Consult your healthcare provider to determine the most appropriate and safe approach for your condition.

Hypothyroidism

Hypothyroidism is a condition in which the thyroid gland does not produce enough thyroid hormones, leading to a range of symptoms, including fatigue, weight gain, dry skin, and more. While medications like levothyroxine are typically prescribed to manage hypothyroidism, there are supportive measures and natural remedies that can help alleviate symptoms and promote thyroid health. These approaches should be used under a healthcare provider's guidance and in conjunction with medical care. Here are some supportive strategies for dealing with hypothyroidism:

Dietary Modifications: Consume a well-balanced diet that includes foods rich in iodine, selenium, and other nutrients essential for thyroid health. Seafood, dairy products, and iodized salt are useful sources of iodine, while selenium can be found in nuts, seeds, and lean meats.

Foods Rich in Tyrosine: Tyrosine is an amino acid that is a precursor to thyroid hormones. Include lean proteins, nuts, and dairy products in your diet.

Cruciferous Vegetables: While cruciferous vegetables like broccoli and cauliflower can interfere with thyroid function when consumed in substantial amounts, cooking or steaming them can help reduce their impact.

Stress Management: Practice stress-reduction techniques like yoga, meditation, or deep breathing exercises, as stress can exacerbate hypothyroid symptoms.

Selenium Supplements: If your diet is deficient in selenium, consider selenium supplements under the guidance of a healthcare provider.

Kelp Supplements: Kelp is a natural source of iodine and is available in supplement form. Use it cautiously and only under the guidance of a healthcare provider to avoid excessive iodine intake.

Coconut Oil: Some people with hypothyroidism have reported improved skin and hair health using coconut oil.

Ashwagandha (Withania somnifera): Ashwagandha is an adaptogenic herb that may help reduce stress and improve overall well-being. Some studies suggest it may have a positive effect on thyroid function. However, research is ongoing, and its role in managing hypothyroidism is not fully established. Consult with a healthcare provider before using it.

Bladderwrack (Fucus vesiculosus): Bladderwrack is a seaweed containing iodine essential for thyroid health. It has been used historically to support thyroid function, especially in cases of iodine deficiency. However, excessive iodine intake can lead to thyroid dysfunction, so it should be used with caution and under the guidance of a healthcare provider.

Lemon Balm (Melissa officinalis): Lemon balm is an herb that may help reduce stress and anxiety, which can be symptoms of hypothyroidism. It is considered safe for use as a tea or supplement.

Immune Support

A robust immune system is crucial for maintaining good health and fighting infections. While no specific "medicinal" plants or herbs can cure or prevent diseases, there are supportive measures and natural remedies that can help strengthen the immune system. These approaches should be used with a healthy lifestyle and not replace medical care when needed. Here are some supportive strategies for immune support:

Balanced Diet: Consume a well-balanced diet rich in fruits, vegetables, whole grains, lean proteins, and healthy fats. These foods provide essential vitamins and minerals that support immune function.

Vitamin C: Foods high in vitamin C, like citrus fruits, strawberries, and bell peppers, can help boost immune health. Vitamin C supplements can also be considered, especially during increased immune stress.

Vitamin D: Adequate levels of vitamin D are essential for immune health. Exposure to sunlight is a natural way to get vitamin D, but supplements can be used if you have a deficiency.

Probiotics: Probiotic supplements or foods like yogurt with live cultures can help maintain a healthy balance of gut bacteria, which plays a crucial role in immune function.

Zinc: Zinc is a mineral that is vital for immune health. Foods rich in zinc include beans, nuts, and whole grains. Zinc supplements can be used if you have a deficiency.

Garlic (Allium sativum): Garlic contains compounds that may have immune-boosting properties. Incorporating garlic into your diet or using garlic supplements may offer immune support.

Echinacea (Echinacea purpurea): Echinacea is an herb that some people use to support the immune system and reduce the severity and duration of colds. It is available as teas, capsules, and tinctures.

Ginger (Zingiber officinale): Ginger has anti-inflammatory and antioxidant properties. Ginger tea or ginger supplements can be used to support immune health.

Herbal Teas: Herbal teas like chamomile, elderberry, and green tea contain compounds that may support immune function. They can be consumed regularly as part of a healthy diet.

Stress Management: Chronic stress can weaken the immune system. Stress-reduction techniques like yoga, meditation, and deep breathing can be beneficial.

Adequate Sleep: Prioritize sleep and aim for 7-9 hours of quality sleep per night to support immune health.

Hydration: Staying well-hydrated is essential for overall health, including the proper functioning of the immune system.

It is important to note that while these supportive measures can contribute to a healthy immune system, no single food or supplement can prevent or cure diseases. Additionally, individual needs vary, and it is advisable to consult with a healthcare provider or registered dietitian before starting any new supplement regimen, especially if you have specific health conditions or are taking medications. Maintaining a balanced and healthy lifestyle with these supportive strategies is the most effective way to promote a strong immune system.

Indigestion

Indigestion, also known as dyspepsia, is a common condition that can cause discomfort and pain in the upper abdomen. There are supportive measures and natural remedies that can help alleviate indigestion symptoms. These approaches should be used in conjunction with a healthy lifestyle. Here are some supportive strategies for managing indigestion:

Ginger (Zingiber officinale): Ginger is known for its digestive properties and may help alleviate indigestion. It can be consumed as ginger tea or added to meals. You can also chew on a small piece of fresh ginger.

Peppermint (Mentha piperita): Peppermint tea or peppermint oil capsules may help relax the gastrointestinal tract muscles and reduce indigestion symptoms.

Chamomile (Matricaria chamomilla): Chamomile tea can have a calming effect on the stomach and may help relieve indigestion.

Fennel (Foeniculum vulgare): Fennel seeds can be chewed or steeped in hot water to make a soothing tea that may aid digestion and relieve indigestion.

Probiotics: Probiotic supplements or foods like yogurt with live cultures can help maintain a healthy balance of gut bacteria and support digestion.

Aloe Vera (Aloe barbadensis miller): Aloe vera juice may help soothe the digestive tract and alleviate indigestion. It is available as a dietary supplement.

Papaya (Carica papaya): Papaya contains enzymes like papain that can aid digestion. Eating fresh papaya or taking papaya enzyme supplements may be beneficial.

Lifestyle Changes: Avoid overeating and consume smaller, more frequent meals to ease digestion. Avoid lying down immediately after eating and maintain an upright position to help prevent indigestion.

Avoid Trigger Foods: Identify and avoid foods that tend to trigger indigestion in your case. Common trigger foods include spicy, greasy, or acidic items, caffeine, and alcohol.

Stress Management: Chronic stress can exacerbate indigestion. Practice stress-reduction techniques like yoga, meditation, and deep breathing to help manage stress.

Adequate Hydration: Drinking enough water throughout the day can aid in digestion.

If you experience severe or persistent indigestion, it is important to consult with a healthcare provider for proper evaluation and treatment. Indigestion can sometimes be a symptom of an underlying medical condition, and it is essential to rule out any serious issues. These natural remedies should not replace medical care for severe or chronic cases.

Insomnia

Insomnia is a common sleep disorder characterized by difficulty falling asleep, staying asleep, or experiencing non-restorative sleep despite having the opportunity to sleep. It can lead to daytime fatigue, irritability, difficulty concentrating, and a reduced overall quality of life. Insomnia can be acute (short-term) or chronic (long-term) and may have various causes, including stress, lifestyle factors, underlying medical conditions, or medications.

Treatment for insomnia often involves a combination of strategies, and it is important to identify and address any underlying causes. Here are some general tips and strategies to manage insomnia:

Sleep Hygiene: Adopt good sleep hygiene practices, including keeping a regular sleep schedule, creating a comfortable sleep environment, and avoiding stimulating activities and electronics before bedtime.

Cognitive-Behavioral Therapy for Insomnia (CBT-I): CBT-I is a structured form of psychotherapy that focuses on changing behaviors and thoughts related to sleep. It has been shown to be effective in treating insomnia.

Stress Management: Stress and anxiety can contribute to insomnia. Relaxation techniques like deep breathing, progressive muscle relaxation, or mindfulness meditation can help reduce stress and improve sleep.

Limit Caffeine and Alcohol: Avoid caffeine and alcohol close to bedtime, as they can disrupt sleep patterns.

Regular Exercise: Regular physical activity can promote better sleep but avoid strenuous exercise close to bedtime.

Bedtime Routine: Establish a calming bedtime routine to signal to your body that it is time to sleep. This might include reading a book, taking a warm bath, or practicing gentle stretching.

Medications: A healthcare provider may sometimes recommend medication to help with insomnia. These should be used under professional guidance and for a limited duration.

The following are some natural remedies that may complement conventional treatments:

Herbal Teas: Certain herbal teas, such as chamomile or valerian root, are thought to have calming properties and may promote relaxation before bedtime.

Lavender (Lavandula spp.): Lavender essential oil or sachets may be used for their soothing scent, which can help create a relaxing sleep environment.

Melatonin: Melatonin is a hormone that helps regulate sleep-wake cycles. Melatonin supplements are available over the counter and can help adjust sleep patterns. Consult with a healthcare provider for appropriate dosages.

Irritable Bowel Syndrome (IBS)

Irritable Bowel Syndrome (IBS) is a common functional gastrointestinal disorder that affects the large intestine (colon). It is characterized by a group of digestive symptoms, varying in severity and duration. Common IBS symptoms include abdominal pain or discomfort, changes in bowel habits (diarrhea, constipation, or both), bloating, and gas. IBS is a chronic condition that can cause considerable discomfort and affect a person's quality of life.

Managing IBS typically involves dietary and lifestyle changes, stress management, and sometimes medications. Here are some general tips and strategies for managing IBS:

Dietary Changes: Many people with IBS find relief by making specific dietary modifications. The Low FODMAP diet is often recommended, which involves avoiding fermentable carbohydrates that can trigger IBS symptoms. Working with a healthcare provider or registered dietitian is crucial for guidance.

Fiber: For some people with IBS, increasing dietary fiber can help regulate bowel movements. Soluble fiber, found in foods like oats and psyllium, is often better tolerated than insoluble fiber.

Probiotics: Probiotic supplements may benefit some individuals with IBS, as they can help balance the gut microbiota. Consult with a healthcare provider for recommendations.

Stress Management: Stress and anxiety can exacerbate IBS symptoms. Practicing relaxation techniques, such as deep breathing, meditation, and mindfulness, can be helpful.

Regular Meals: Eating and not skipping regular meals can help regulate digestive patterns.

Hydration:
Staying well-hydrated is important, as insufficient fluid intake can lead to constipation or worsening symptoms.

Medications: A healthcare provider may sometimes prescribe medications to manage specific symptoms. These may include antispasmodic drugs for abdominal pain, antidiarrheal medications, or medications that affect gut motility.

Lifestyle Changes: Regular physical activity and a good sleep routine can contribute to overall well-being and may help manage IBS symptoms.

Some natural remedies and dietary modifications may be considered.

Peppermint (Mentha × piperita): Peppermint oil capsules have been found to help relieve symptoms of IBS, particularly abdominal pain, and bloating.

Ginger (Zingiber officinale): Ginger may help alleviate nausea and reduce inflammation in the gut.

Chamomile (Matricaria chamomilla): Chamomile tea may have anti-inflammatory and calming properties.

Aloe Vera (Aloe barbadensis miller): Aloe vera juice or supplements have been used traditionally to soothe gastrointestinal discomfort.

Natural remedies for IBS should be used with caution and under the guidance of a healthcare provider. It is important to consult a healthcare professional for an accurate diagnosis and a personalized treatment plan. IBS is a complex condition, and the specific management approach can vary from person to person. Natural remedies may complement traditional treatments but should not replace evidence-based medical care when necessary.

Joint Health

Joint health refers to the condition and well-being of the joints in your body, which are crucial for mobility and overall quality of life. Maintaining joint health prevents joint pain, stiffness, and osteoarthritis. Several lifestyle practices and natural supplements may support joint health and relieve discomfort:

Exercise: Regular physical activity, such as low-impact exercises, strength training, and flexibility exercises, can help maintain joint health, improve range of motion, and reduce the risk of joint problems.

Weight Management: Maintaining a healthy weight can reduce stress on the joints, particularly those in the lower body, such as the knees and hips.

Balanced Diet: A diet rich in anti-inflammatory foods, such as fatty fish (e.g., salmon, mackerel), colorful fruits and vegetables, and whole grains, may help reduce inflammation and support joint health.

Supplements: Some natural supplements have been studied for their potential benefits in promoting joint health. These include

Glucosamine and Chondroitin: These compounds are naturally found in cartilage and are available as supplements. Some people take them to support joint health, although their effectiveness is still a topic of research.

Turmeric (Curcuma longa): Turmeric is a spice that contains curcumin, known for its anti-inflammatory properties. Some people take curcumin supplements for joint pain relief.

Omega-3 Fatty Acids: In fish oil and certain seeds and nuts, omega-3 fatty acids may help reduce joint inflammation.

Boswellia (Boswellia serrata): Extracted from the resin of Boswellia trees, boswellia supplements are used by some people to manage joint pain and inflammation.

MSM (Methylsulfonylmethane): MSM is a sulfur-containing compound that may support joint health. It is available in supplement form.

Heat and Cold Therapy: Applying heat or cold to the affected joint temporarily relieves pain and stiffness.

Rest and Joint Protection: Avoid overusing or overloading your joints. Proper body mechanics and joint protection techniques can help prevent further joint damage.

Orthopedic Supports: Depending on the type and location of joint issues, orthopedic supports like braces or splints may be helpful. Consult a healthcare provider for recommendations.

Joint Inflammation

Joint inflammation refers to the swelling, redness, and discomfort in the joints due to an immune response, injury, or underlying medical condition. Joint inflammation can lead to pain, stiffness, and reduced mobility. While there are no specific medicinal plants, mushrooms, or trees grown in the US that are medically proven to "treat" joint inflammation, several lifestyle practices, and natural supplements may help manage inflammation and support joint health:

Anti-Inflammatory Diet: Consuming a diet rich in anti-inflammatory foods, such as fatty fish, colorful fruits and vegetables, whole grains, and herbs like turmeric, may help reduce joint inflammation.

Omega-3 Fatty Acids: Omega-3 fatty acids found in fish oil and certain plant sources have anti-inflammatory properties. Incorporating these into your diet or taking supplements can help manage inflammation.

Turmeric (Curcuma longa): Turmeric contains curcumin, a compound with potent anti-inflammatory properties. Some people take curcumin supplements to reduce inflammation and joint pain.

Ginger (Zingiber officinale): Ginger has natural anti-inflammatory properties and may help alleviate joint pain and stiffness.

Boswellia (Boswellia serrata): Boswellia supplements, derived from the resin of Boswellia trees, are used by some people to manage inflammation and joint pain.

MSM (Methylsulfonylmethane): MSM is a sulfur-containing compound that may support joint health and help manage inflammation. It is available in supplement form.

Heat and Cold Therapy: Applying heat or cold to the inflamed joint temporarily relieves pain and swelling.

Regular Exercise: Regular physical activity can help maintain joint health and reduce inflammation. Low-impact exercises, strength training, and flexibility exercises can be beneficial.

Weight Management: Maintaining a healthy weight can reduce joint stress and help manage inflammation.

Supplements: Some natural supplements, like glucosamine and chondroitin, have been studied for their potential benefits in promoting joint health and reducing inflammation. Their effectiveness varies from person to person.

It is essential to consult with a healthcare provider before using any natural supplements or making significant dietary changes, especially if you are taking medications or have underlying health conditions. Joint inflammation management should be individualized to your specific condition and needs, and natural remedies should complement conventional treatments when necessary. If you are experiencing persistent joint inflammation or suspect an underlying joint condition, it is important to consult with a healthcare provider for a proper diagnosis and treatment plan.

Kidney Disorders

Kidney disorders refer to a wide range of medical conditions that affect the kidneys, two bean-shaped organs in the back of the abdomen. The kidneys filter waste and excess substances from the blood, regulate blood pressure, balance electrolytes, and produce hormones.

Kidney disorders can vary in severity, including chronic kidney disease (CKD), kidney stones, and infections. Management of kidney disorders depends on the specific condition and its underlying causes. Consulting with a healthcare provider for a proper diagnosis and treatment plan is important. While there are no specific medicinal plants, mushrooms, or trees grown in the US that are medically proven to "treat" kidney disorders, several general lifestyle practices, and dietary considerations can promote kidney health and support overall well-being:

Hydration: Staying well-hydrated is essential for kidney health. Drinking adequate water helps flush waste and toxins from the body.

Balanced Diet: A diet low in salt and saturated fats and rich in fruits, vegetables, whole grains, and lean proteins can support overall health, including kidney health.

Blood Pressure Management: High blood pressure can harm the kidneys. If you have high blood pressure, work with your healthcare provider to manage it effectively.

Diabetes Management: Uncontrolled diabetes can also harm the kidneys. Proper management of diabetes is important for kidney health.

Regular Exercise: Regular physical activity can support overall health, including cardiovascular health, which is important for kidney function.

Dandelion (Taraxacum officinale): Dandelion is known for its diuretic (increases urine production) properties, which may help flush waste and excess bodily fluids. This can be beneficial for individuals with mild fluid retention. Dandelion contains antioxidants, which can help protect the kidneys from oxidative stress. Dandelion leaves are a useful source of vitamins (like A, C, and K) and minerals (like potassium), which can support overall health.
Precautions: Dandelion may interact with certain medications or worsen symptoms in people with kidney stones. It is important to consult a healthcare provider before using dandelion as a remedy, especially if you have kidney issues or are taking medications.

Horsetail (Equisetum arvense): Horsetail also has diuretic properties that may help increase urine output and potentially assist in eliminating waste from the kidneys. Horsetail is rich in silica, which can support tissue health and repair. Precautions: Horsetail contains a compound called thiaminase, which can interfere with the absorption of thiamine (vitamin B1). Excessive use of horsetail may lead to thiamine deficiency. It is important to use horsetail under the guidance of a healthcare provider and for limited durations.

Avoiding Overuse of Over-the-Counter Pain Relievers: Some non-prescription pain relievers, such as nonsteroidal anti-inflammatory drugs (NSAIDs), can harm the kidneys when used excessively.

Limiting Alcohol: Excessive alcohol consumption can harm kidney health.

Smoking Cessation: Smoking is harmful to the kidneys and overall health. Quitting smoking can benefit your kidneys and reduce the risk of various health issues.

It is important to note that specific kidney disorders may require specialized medical treatment, and natural remedies should be used with caution and in consultation with a healthcare provider. Kidney health management should be individualized to your specific condition and needs. Natural remedies should complement conventional treatments when necessary, and any changes to your treatment plan should be made in consultation with a healthcare provider.

Kidney Stones

Kidney stones are solid, pebble-like substances that form in the kidneys when elevated levels of certain minerals and salts are in your urine. These minerals can crystallize and accumulate to create stones, which can be painful and may block the urinary tract. Kidney stones can vary in size and composition, and they can cause symptoms such as severe pain, blood in the urine, and urinary tract infections.

Management of kidney stones typically depends on the size, type, and location of the stones and the severity of symptoms. Some stones may pass independently, while others may require medical intervention. Consulting with a healthcare provider for proper diagnosis and treatment is essential. Here are some general tips and dietary considerations that may help reduce the risk of kidney stone formation and support kidney health:

Hydration: Staying well-hydrated is crucial. Drinking enough water can help dilute urine and prevent the accumulation of minerals that can lead to stone formation.

Dietary Changes: Dietary modifications may be recommended depending on the type of kidney stones you are prone to. For example, reducing high-oxalate foods like spinach, beets, and chocolate may be advised if you have calcium oxalate stones.

Limit Sodium: Reducing dietary sodium (salt) intake can help lower the risk of stone formation, particularly for individuals prone to calcium-containing stones.

Calcium Intake: Adequate dietary calcium may benefit some individuals, as it can bind to oxalate and reduce the risk of stone formation. Consult with a healthcare provider for specific recommendations.

Citrate: Citrate in citrus fruits can help prevent stone formation. Consuming citrus fruits or potassium citrate supplements may be recommended.

Moderate Protein Intake: Excessive protein intake can produce substances that increase the risk of stone formation.

Medications: In some cases, healthcare providers may prescribe medications to manage the underlying causes of kidney stone formation.

Herbal teas or supplements: These are sometimes used to help prevent or manage kidney stones. For example, chanca piedra (Phyllanthus niruri) is a traditional herbal remedy used in some cultures for its potential to break down kidney stones and help them pass more easily. It is important to consult with a healthcare provider before using such remedies, especially if you have existing kidney issues or are taking medications.

Kidney stone management should be individualized to your specific condition and needs, and natural remedies should complement, not replace, conventional treatments when necessary. If you experience symptoms of kidney stones, such as severe pain, blood in the urine, or difficulty urinating, seek immediate medical attention.

Liver Disorders

Liver disorders encompass a wide range of conditions that affect the liver, a vital organ responsible for processing nutrients, removing toxins, producing proteins, and regulating metabolism. Liver disorders can vary in severity including hepatitis, cirrhosis, fatty liver disease, liver cancer, and more. Management of liver disorders depends on the specific condition and its underlying causes. Consulting with a healthcare provider for a proper diagnosis and treatment plan is important.

Several general lifestyle practices and dietary considerations can promote liver health and support overall well-being:

Moderate Alcohol Consumption: Excessive alcohol intake can harm the liver. If you consume alcohol, do so in moderation or consider abstaining.

Healthy Diet: A balanced diet is low in saturated fats and added sugars and rich in fruits, vegetables, whole grains, and lean proteins can support overall health, including liver health.

Weight Management: Maintaining a healthy weight is important, as obesity can contribute to non-alcoholic fatty liver disease (NAFLD).

Hepatitis Vaccination: Vaccination can protect against hepatitis A and hepatitis B, viral infections that can damage the liver. Regular Exercise: Regular physical activity can support overall health, including cardiovascular health, which is important for liver function.

Medication Management: If you are on medications that may affect the liver, follow your healthcare provider's instructions, and attend regular check-ups.

Liver-Friendly Foods: Certain foods, like garlic (Allium sativum), grapefruit, beets, dandelion (Taraxacum officinale), and milk thistle (Silybum marianum), are thought to support liver health. Including them in your diet can be beneficial.

Milk Thistle (Silybum marianum): Milk thistle has been traditionally used to support liver health. It contains a compound called silymarin, believed to have antioxidant and anti-inflammatory properties that may help protect the liver. Dandelion is known for its diuretic properties and may aid in detoxification processes.

It is important to consult with a healthcare provider before making significant dietary changes or using natural supplements, especially if you have liver issues or are taking medications. Liver health management should be individualized to your specific condition and needs, and natural remedies should complement, not replace, conventional treatments when necessary.

Suppose you are experiencing symptoms of liver disorders, such as jaundice (yellowing of the skin or eyes), abdominal pain, unexplained weight loss, or changes in urine or stool color. In that case, consulting with a healthcare provider for a proper diagnosis and treatment plan is crucial in that case. Liver disorders can have profound consequences, and early intervention is often key to effective management.

Memory and Cognitive Function

Memory and cognitive function are essential to our well-being. Cognitive function encompasses various mental processes, including memory, attention, problem-solving, and reasoning. Maintaining good cognitive function is vital for daily activities and quality of life. Several general lifestyle practices and dietary considerations may support cognitive health and memory.

Healthy Diet: A balanced diet that includes various fruits, vegetables, whole grains, lean proteins, and healthy fats provides essential nutrients for brain health. Foods rich in antioxidants, such as berries, and omega-3 fatty acids, like fatty fish, may support cognitive function.

Hydration: Staying well-hydrated is crucial for optimal brain function. Dehydration can impair cognitive performance.

Regular Physical Activity: Exercise promotes blood flow and oxygen delivery to the brain, improving cognitive function and memory.

Adequate Sleep: Quality sleep is essential for memory consolidation and overall cognitive performance. Aim for 7-9 hours of sleep per night.

Mental Stimulation: Engage in activities that challenge your brain, such as puzzles, learning new skills, or playing musical instruments.

Social Interaction: Socializing and maintaining strong social connections can positively impact cognitive function.

Chronic stress can negatively affect memory and cognitive function. Practice stress-reduction techniques, such as meditation, mindfulness, or relaxation exercises.

Limit Alcohol: Excessive alcohol consumption can impair memory and cognitive function. If you drink alcohol, do so in moderation.

Avoid Smoking: Smoking can harm blood vessels and reduce oxygen flow to the brain, potentially affecting cognitive function.

Medication Management: Some medications can impact cognitive function. Discuss any concerns with your healthcare provider.

Some commonly mentioned supplements for cognitive health include:

Ginkgo Biloba (Ginkgo biloba): It is believed to improve blood flow to the brain.

Bacopa (Bacopa monnieri): This herb is thought to enhance memory and cognitive function.

Ginseng (Panax quinquefolius): Some studies suggest it may have cognitive-enhancing effects.

Menopause Symptoms

Menopause Symptoms and Herbal Remedies:

Menopause is a natural transition in a woman's life marked by hormonal changes, particularly a decrease in estrogen. While some women may not experience significant symptoms, others may find the transition challenging. Some women have used herbal remedies to help alleviate menopause symptoms. Remember that the effectiveness of herbal remedies can vary among individuals, and it is essential to consult with a healthcare provider before using them, especially if you have any underlying health conditions or are taking medications. Here are some herbal remedies for managing menopause symptoms:

Black Cohosh (Cimicifuga racemosa).

Black cohosh is a commonly used herbal remedy for menopausal symptoms. It is believed to have mild estrogen-like effects that may help alleviate hot flashes, mood swings, and sleep disturbances. Some studies suggest it can be effective, but more research is needed.

Red Clover (Trifolium pratense): Red clover contains phytoestrogens, plant compounds that can mimic the effects of estrogen in the body. These compounds may help relieve hot flashes and night sweats. While some studies have shown promise, results are mixed.

Soy Products: Soy contains isoflavones, another type of phytoestrogen. Consuming soy products like tofu and soy milk may help manage hot flashes and mood changes. Soy is a staple in many Asian diets; some studies suggest it may be effective.

Dong Quai (Angelica sinensis): Dong Quai is a traditional Chinese herb that relieves menopausal symptoms such as hot flashes and mood swings. However, more research is needed to confirm its effectiveness.

Evening Primrose Oil: Evening primrose oil, rich in gamma-linolenic acid, is believed to help with mood swings and breast tenderness during menopause. Its efficacy is still under investigation.

Chasteberry (Vitex agnus-castus): Chasteberry may help with mood changes, especially irritability and mood swings, but it is less commonly used for other menopausal symptoms.

Ginseng (Panax quinquefolius): Ginseng may offer benefits for mood and cognitive function during menopause. American ginseng (Panax quinquefolius) and Asian ginseng (Panax ginseng) are used.

St. John's Wort (Hypericum perforatum): St. John's wort is sometimes used for mood-related symptoms like irritability and mild depression. However, it can interact with medications, so it should be used cautiously and under a healthcare provider's guidance.

Consulting with a healthcare provider or herbalist who is knowledgeable about the use of herbs during menopause is advisable. They can help determine which remedies, if any, are safe and appropriate for your specific needs.

Menstrual Disorders

Menstrual disorders encompass various conditions that can disrupt a woman's menstrual cycle, leading to irregularity, heavy bleeding, painful menstruation, or even the absence of periods. While pharmaceutical and medical treatments are available, many women seek solace in natural herbal remedies to alleviate symptoms and promote menstrual health.

Menstrual Irregularities: Herbal remedies like chasteberry (Vitex agnus-castus) are known for balancing hormones and promoting regular menstruation. This herb may help address irregular cycles and establish a more predictable pattern.

Amenorrhea: In cases of secondary amenorrhea, where periods have ceased, herbs like black cohosh (Actaea racemosa) are believed to address hormonal imbalances. Black cohosh may support the restoration of a regular menstrual cycle.

Dysmenorrhea (Menstrual Cramps): Herbal teas or supplements containing ingredients such as ginger, chamomile, or cramp bark (Viburnum opulus) are renowned for their pain-relieving properties. These herbs may help reduce the intensity of menstrual cramps and alleviate discomfort.

Menorrhagia (Heavy Bleeding): Herbs with astringent qualities, like yarrow (Achillea millefolium) and shepherd's purse (Capsella bursa-pastoris), are often used to control excessive menstrual bleeding. These herbs may help to moderate-heavy flow.

Polycystic Ovary Syndrome (PCOS): Spearmint tea and saw palmetto are believed to have anti-androgenic properties, which may help manage PCOS symptoms by reducing excessive hair growth and acne.

Premenstrual Syndrome (PMS): Supplements like evening primrose oil (Oenothera biennis) or borage oil can alleviate mood swings and breast tenderness, common symptoms associated with PMS.

Chasteberry (Vitex agnus-castus): Chasteberry is renowned for its hormone-regulating properties. This herb may help balance the pituitary gland's function, reducing prolactin levels and restoring regular menstruation. It is a valuable remedy for addressing irregular menstrual cycles.

Black Cohosh (Actaea racemosa): Black cohosh has been traditionally used to address hormonal imbalances and alleviate symptoms associated with menopause and menstruation. It may help reduce cramping, regulate menstruation, and ease mood swings.

Cramp Bark (Viburnum opulus): Cramp bark is a natural muscle relaxant. It can be beneficial for relieving severe menstrual cramps, as it eases muscle tension in the uterine area. This herb can significantly reduce the intensity of cramping.

Yarrow (Achillea millefolium): Yarrow is an astringent herb that may help manage heavy menstrual bleeding. It can help constrict blood vessels and reduce excessive flow, leading to more manageable menstruation.

Shepherd's Purse (Capsella bursa-pastoris): Shepherd's purse is another excellent herb for controlling heavy bleeding. It possesses hemostatic properties, which can help stop bleeding by promoting clot formation.

Ginger (Zingiber officinale): Ginger is well-known for its anti-inflammatory and pain-relieving properties. It can be used to alleviate menstrual cramps, reducing pain and discomfort.

Chamomile (Matricaria chamomilla): Chamomile is often used in herbal teas to help relax the mind and body, making it a valuable choice for reducing stress and tension associated with menstruation.

Evening Primrose Oil (Oenothera biennis): Evening primrose oil contains gamma-linolenic acid, which may help alleviate breast tenderness and mood swings associated with PMS.

Borage oil is a source of essential fatty acids and can alleviate mood swings, breast tenderness, and other PMS symptoms.

These natural herbal remedies are considered safe and offer an integrated approach to managing menstrual disorders. However, it is essential to recognize that individual responses to herbs can vary, and not all remedies are universally effective. Consulting with an herbalist or healthcare provider experienced in botanical medicine is prudent. They can assist in selecting the right herbs, recommend appropriate dosages, and discuss potential interactions with other medications or health conditions.

Alongside herbal remedies, a balanced lifestyle with a nutritious diet, regular exercise, and effective stress management is vital for promoting overall menstrual health. Consult your doctor if you experience severe or debilitating menstrual symptoms or have concerns about your condition.

Menstrual Irregularities

Menstrual irregularities refer to variations or abnormalities in the timing, frequency, or flow of a woman's menstrual cycle. These irregularities can include

Amenorrhea and the absence of menstrual periods, which can be classified as primary (never having had a period by age 16) or secondary (absence of periods for at least three months in a woman who previously had regular cycles).

Oligomenorrhea: Infrequent periods, with cycles lasting longer than 35 days.

Poly menorrhea: Frequent periods with cycles shorter than 21 days.

Menorrhagia: Excessively heavy menstrual bleeding, often accompanied by clots, lasts longer than seven days.

Metrorrhagia: Irregular bleeding or spotting between periods.

Dysmenorrhea: Painful menstruation, often accompanied by severe cramps.

Anovulation: A condition where an egg is not released from the ovaries during a menstrual cycle.

Hypomenorrhea: Light menstrual flow, where periods produce significantly less blood than usual.

Hypermenorrhea: Abnormally heavy menstrual flow, but not to the extent of menorrhagia.

Causes of Menstrual Irregularities:

Several factors can contribute to menstrual irregularities:

Hormonal Imbalances: Fluctuations in estrogen and progesterone levels can disrupt the menstrual cycle.

Stress: High-stress levels can affect the hypothalamus, impacting the production of hormones that regulate the menstrual cycle.

Polycystic Ovary Syndrome (PCOS): A common condition that can lead to irregular periods, amenorrhea, and anovulation.

Thyroid Disorders: Thyroid imbalances can affect hormone regulation, leading to irregular menstrual.

Uterine Conditions: Fibroids, polyps, or endometriosis can affect the uterine lining and menstrual flow.

Eating Disorders: Anorexia and bulimia can disrupt the menstrual cycle due to extreme weight loss.

Excessive Exercise: Intense physical activity can lead to amenorrhea, especially when combined with inadequate calorie intake.

Perimenopause: The transition to menopause (perimenopause) often comes with irregular periods.

Treatment and Management: The approach to treating and managing menstrual irregularities depends on the underlying cause. Treatment options may include

Hormonal Birth Control: This can help regulate the menstrual cycle and alleviate symptoms.

Lifestyle Modifications: Stress management, a balanced diet, and regular exercise can support menstrual health.

Medications: Non-prescription pain relievers like ibuprofen can help manage menstrual cramps.

Hormone Therapy: Hormone therapy can be prescribed to address hormonal imbalances.

Chasteberry (Vitex agnus-castus): Chasteberry is renowned for its hormone-regulating properties. This herb may help balance the pituitary gland's function, reducing prolactin levels and restoring regular menstruation. It is a valuable remedy for addressing irregular menstrual cycles.

Black Cohosh (Actaea racemosa): Black cohosh has been traditionally used to address hormonal imbalances and alleviate symptoms associated with menopause and menstruation. It may help reduce cramping, regulate menstruation, and ease mood swings.

Cramp Bark (Viburnum opulus): Cramp bark is a natural muscle relaxant. It can be beneficial for relieving severe menstrual cramps, as it eases muscle tension in the uterine area. This herb can significantly reduce the intensity of cramping.

Yarrow (Achillea millefolium): Yarrow is an astringent herb that may help manage heavy menstrual bleeding. It can help constrict blood vessels and reduce excessive flow, leading to more manageable menstruation.

Shepherd's Purse (Capsella bursa-pastoris): Shepherd's purse is another excellent herb for controlling heavy bleeding. It possesses hemostatic properties, which can help stop bleeding by promoting clot formation.

Ginger (Zingiber officinale): Ginger is well-known for its anti-inflammatory and pain-relieving properties. It can be used to alleviate menstrual cramps, reducing pain and discomfort.

Chamomile (Matricaria chamomilla): Chamomile is often used in herbal teas to help relax the mind and body, making it a valuable choice for reducing stress and tension associated with menstruation.

Evening Primrose Oil (Oenothera biennis): Evening primrose oil contains gamma-linolenic acid, which may help alleviate breast tenderness and mood swings associated with PMS.

Borage Oil (Borago officinalis): Borage oil is a source of essential fatty acids and can alleviate mood swings, breast tenderness, and other PMS symptoms.

Menstrual Pain

Menstrual pain, also known as dysmenorrhea, is a common discomfort experienced by many women during their menstrual cycles. This pain is typically characterized by cramping in the lower abdomen, although it can radiate to the lower back and thighs. Menstrual pain can range from mild to severe and may be accompanied by other symptoms such as nausea, headache, and diarrhea.

There are two types of menstrual pain:

Primary Dysmenorrhea: This is the most common type of menstrual pain and typically occurs without an underlying medical condition. It usually begins a day or two before menstruation and lasts two to four days. The contraction of the uterine muscles causes pain as they expel the uterine lining. It often improves with age and after childbirth.

Secondary Dysmenorrhea: This type of menstrual pain is associated with an underlying medical condition, such as endometriosis, fibroids, or pelvic inflammatory disease. The pain is usually more severe and can begin earlier in the menstrual cycle. Treating the underlying condition is often necessary to alleviate the pain.

There are several ways to manage and alleviate menstrual pain:

Over-the-Counter Pain Relievers: Non-prescription pain relievers such as ibuprofen (Advil), naproxen (Aleve), or aspirin can help reduce menstrual cramps and discomfort.

Prescription Medications: For severe menstrual pain, a healthcare provider may prescribe stronger pain relievers or hormonal medications like birth control pills, which can regulate the menstrual cycle and reduce pain.

Heat Therapy: Applying a heating pad or warm water bottle to the lower abdomen can help relax the uterine muscles and relieve cramps.

Dietary Changes: Reducing salt, caffeine, and alcohol intake can help minimize bloating and fluid retention. A diet rich in fruits, vegetables, and whole grains may also help.

Exercise: Regular physical activity, especially exercises focusing on the pelvic area, like yoga or stretching, can help reduce menstrual pain.

Relaxation Techniques: Stress management, relaxation, and deep breathing exercises can help relax the body and reduce pain.

Herbal Remedies: Some women relieve menstrual pain through herbal remedies like ginger, chamomile, and cramp bark. These herbs can be consumed as teas or supplements.

Acupuncture and Acupressure: Some women report relief from menstrual pain through acupuncture or acupressure sessions, which focus on stimulating specific points in the body.

Ginger (Zingiber officinale): Ginger is well-known for its anti-inflammatory and pain-relieving properties. It can be used to alleviate menstrual cramps, reducing pain and discomfort.

Chamomile (Matricaria chamomilla): Chamomile is often used in herbal teas to help relax the mind and body, making it a valuable choice for reducing stress and tension associated with menstruation.

Cramp Bark (Viburnum opulus): Cramp bark is a natural muscle relaxant. It can be beneficial for relieving severe menstrual cramps, as it eases muscle tension in the uterine area. This herb can significantly reduce the intensity of cramping.

It is essential to consult with a healthcare provider if you experience severe or debilitating menstrual pain, as this may be a sign of an underlying condition that needs to be addressed. They can accurately diagnose and recommend the most appropriate treatment for your situation.

Migraines

Migraines, known for their debilitating throbbing pain, often accompanied by nausea, vomiting, and sensitivity to light and sound, can significantly disrupt daily life. While prescription and over-the-counter medications are commonly used to manage migraines, some individuals use natural herbal remedies to complement traditional treatments. Here, we explore some of these herbal remedies, their potential benefits, and how they can aid in managing migraines:

Feverfew (Tanacetum parthenium): Feverfew is one of the most widely recognized herbal remedies for migraines. It is believed to reduce the frequency and severity of migraine attacks. Its anti-inflammatory and vasodilatory properties may help ease the constriction of blood vessels in the head, a common feature of migraines.

Butterbur (Petasites hybridus): Butterbur is another herbal remedy frequently used to manage migraines. Its active compounds, petasins, have anti-inflammatory and muscle-relaxant properties. These properties may help alleviate the constriction of blood vessels in the brain and reduce migraine-related pain.

Ginger (Zingiber officinale): Ginger has anti-inflammatory properties that may help reduce migraine pain and nausea. It can be consumed in various forms, such as ginger tea or supplements.

Riboflavin (Vitamin B2): Riboflavin, or vitamin B2, has shown promise in reducing the frequency and severity of migraines when taken as a supplement. It is involved in producing cellular energy and may have a role in regulating blood vessel function.

Peppermint (Mentha × piperita): Peppermint oil, applied topically or inhaled, may help alleviate migraine-related symptoms, particularly nausea, and sensitivity to odors. The soothing aroma and menthol in peppermint can provide relief.

Lavender (Lavandula angustifolia): Lavender essential oil, inhaled or used in aromatherapy, may help relax and reduce stress and anxiety, which can be migraine triggers for some individuals.

Valerian (Valeriana officinalis): Valerian root is known for its calming and sedative properties. It can benefit those whose migraines are triggered or exacerbated by stress or anxiety.

Passionflower (Passiflora incarnata): Passionflower is another herb with sedative properties that can promote relaxation and reduce stress, potentially lessening the occurrence of stress-induced migraines.

It is important to note that while many people find relief from migraines using these herbal remedies, individual responses can vary. Consultation with an herbalist or healthcare provider experienced in botanical medicine is advisable to determine the right herbs, dosages, and potential interactions with other medications or health conditions.

These natural herbal remedies can be part of a comprehensive approach to managing migraines, including lifestyle modifications, stress management, and prescription medications for severe cases.

Morning Sickness (Pregnancy-Related Nausea)

Morning sickness, also known as pregnancy-related nausea, is a common condition that affects many pregnant women during the first trimester of pregnancy. It is characterized by feelings of nausea and vomiting, which can occur at any time of the day, not just in the morning. While it can be uncomfortable, morning sickness is usually considered a normal part of pregnancy and typically improves as the pregnancy progresses.

Key aspects of morning sickness include

Nausea: Expectant mothers with morning sickness often experience mild to moderate nausea, which may be persistent or intermittent.

Vomiting: Some women may vomit due to the intensity of nausea.

Sensitivity to Smells: Many pregnant women become more sensitive to certain odors and may find that strong or unpleasant smells trigger nausea.

Taste Changes: Some foods and drinks may taste different to pregnant women, and this can contribute to feelings of nausea.

Trigger Factors: Morning sickness can be triggered by a range of factors, including hormonal changes, increased blood flow to the abdominal area, and psychological factors.

Management and relief from morning sickness often involve the following strategies:

Dietary Modifications: Eating smaller, more frequent meals can help regulate blood sugar levels and reduce the likelihood of nausea. It is also essential to stay hydrated by sipping fluids throughout the day.

Ginger (Zingiber officinale): Ginger is a natural remedy that may help alleviate nausea. It can be consumed in various forms, such as ginger tea, candies, or supplements.

Acupressure Bands: Wristbands designed to stimulate acupressure points may help some women reduce feelings of nausea.

Lemon Balm (Melissa officinalis) and Peppermint (Mentha × piperita): The scents of lemon or peppermint essential oils or lozenges can be soothing and may relieve nausea.

Avoiding Trigger Odors: Identifying and avoiding odors or foods that trigger nausea is crucial. Adequate ventilation and fresh air can also help.

Rest and Stress Management: Fatigue and stress can exacerbate morning sickness. Adequate rest and stress-reduction techniques can help alleviate symptoms.

Vitamin B6: In some cases, healthcare providers may recommend vitamin B6 supplements to manage nausea.

Prescription Medications: In severe cases, prescription medications may be prescribed to manage morning sickness.

Motion Sickness

Motion sickness is a common condition when the brain receives conflicting signals from the senses, leading to symptoms like nausea, dizziness, and occasionally vomiting. This often occurs during travel, such as car rides, boat trips, or air travel. Managing motion sickness involves several strategies, including using natural remedies to alleviate symptoms. Here are some key elements of motion sickness management, incorporating two natural remedies—ginger and peppermint:

Nausea and Discomfort. The hallmark of motion sickness is nausea, ranging from mild discomfort to severe queasiness.

Vomiting: In more severe cases, vomiting may add to the distress.

Dizziness: Dizziness and a sense of instability are common during motion sickness.

Visual-Body Mismatch: Motion sickness often results from a disparity between what the eyes perceive and what the inner ear senses, causing sensory confusion.

Management Strategies:

Position and Stability: Select a stable position, such as the front seat in a car or a seat over the wing of an airplane, to minimize motion sensations.

Horizon Fixation: Gazing at the horizon can help align visual and inner ear cues, reducing the risk of motion sickness.

Ginger (Zingiber officinale): Ginger, renowned for its anti-nausea properties, can be highly effective. Whether consumed as ginger tea, candies, or supplements, it has been shown to ease motion sickness symptoms.

Peppermint (Mentha × piperita): Peppermint's soothing aroma and menthol content can help alleviate nausea and relieve motion sickness. Peppermint lozenges or inhaling peppermint essential oil can be beneficial.

Avoid Reading and Screens: Reading, watching movies, or using electronic devices during travel can exacerbate motion sickness. It is advisable to focus on a stationary point outside the vehicle.

Acupressure Bands: Some individuals find relief from motion sickness using wristbands designed to stimulate acupressure points.

Medications:
Over the counter or prescription medications, such as antihistamines, are available for more severe cases of motion sickness.

Habituation:
Many individuals become less susceptible to motion sickness as they become more accustomed to travel experiences.

In severe symptoms that significantly disrupt daily activities, consulting with a healthcare provider can lead to effective management through medications or treatments tailored to individual needs.

Multiple Sclerosis

Multiple sclerosis is a chronic autoimmune neurological condition affecting the central nervous system, characterized by inflammation and damage to the myelin sheath that protects nerve fibers. While there is no cure for MS, various treatment options can help manage it and its symptoms. Some individuals with MS turn to natural supplements to complement their treatment strategies, and two such supplements are Turmeric (Curcuma longa) and Omega-3 Fatty Acids (from fish).

Key aspects of MS management and treatment:

Symptoms:
MS symptoms can be varied, including fatigue, numbness, weakness, coordination difficulties, muscle spasms, vision problems, and cognitive challenges.

Types of MS: MS can manifest in different forms, including Relapsing-Remitting MS (RRMS), Secondary Progressive MS (SPMS), and Primary Progressive MS (PPMS), each with distinct progression patterns.

Disease-Modifying Therapies: Medications known as disease-modifying therapies can help slow down the progression of the disease and manage relapses.

Symptomatic Treatment: Medications and therapies alleviate specific symptoms such as pain, muscle spasms, and fatigue.

Physical and Occupational Therapy: Rehabilitation therapies help individuals improve mobility and daily living skills.

Healthy Lifestyle: Regular exercise, a balanced diet, and stress management are crucial in managing symptoms and overall well-being.

Supportive Devices: Assistive devices like canes and mobility aids assist in maintaining independence.

Turmeric (Curcuma longa): Turmeric contains an active compound called curcumin, known for its anti-inflammatory and antioxidant properties. It can reduce inflammation and help alleviate some of the symptoms associated with MS. Individuals with MS may incorporate turmeric into their diet or take curcumin supplements. Still, it is essential to consult with a healthcare provider to ensure it is safe and effective for their situation.

Omega-3 Fatty Acids (from fish): Omega-3 fatty acids, primarily found in fatty fish like salmon, mackerel, and trout, are known for their anti-inflammatory properties. Some studies suggest that omega-3 supplementation may help reduce inflammation and potentially benefit individuals with MS. Omega-3 supplements, when taken in appropriate doses, can be a part of a comprehensive treatment plan when taken in appropriate doses.

Alternative and Complementary Therapies: Some individuals explore complementary therapies like acupuncture, yoga, or mindfulness to manage symptoms and improve their quality of life.

Emotional and Psychological Support: Counseling and support groups provide crucial emotional and psychological support in coping with the challenges of living with MS.

It is important to emphasize that supplements and alternative treatments should be approached with caution and under the guidance of a healthcare provider, as their effectiveness and safety can vary among individuals. MS management should be individualized to address each patient's needs and improve their quality of life.

Muscle Pain

Muscle pain, often caused by overuse, tension, or injury, can be alleviated using various natural remedies, including Arnica (Arnica montana) and Cayenne Pepper (Capsicum annuum).

Causes: Muscle pain can result from a range of factors, including muscle strain, overuse, tension, or injury.

Key aspects of muscle pain relief and management:

Resting the affected muscle is often the initial step in recovery, as it allows the muscle to heal.

Heat and Cold Therapy: Applying heat (such as warm compresses) or cold (ice packs) can help reduce inflammation and relieve muscle pain. The choice between heat and cold depends on the type of injury.

Stretching and Exercise: Gentle stretching exercises can help improve flexibility and alleviate muscle tension. Physical therapy or targeted exercises may be recommended for specific conditions.

Hydration: Staying well-hydrated is essential for muscle health. Dehydration can lead to muscle cramps and pain.

Massage:
Therapeutic massage can help relax and alleviate tense muscles, improving blood flow and reducing pain.

Arnica (Arnica montana): Arnica is a well-known natural remedy for muscle pain. Its active compounds have anti-inflammatory and analgesic properties, which can help reduce pain and inflammation when applied topically as an arnica cream or gel. Following usage instructions is important and avoiding applying it to broken skin.

Cayenne Pepper (Capsicum annuum): Cayenne pepper contains capsaicin, which can reduce pain by desensitizing pain receptors in the affected area. Topical creams or ointments containing capsaicin are available and can provide relief when applied to sore muscles.

Over-the-Counter Pain Relievers: Non-prescription pain relievers, such as ibuprofen or acetaminophen, can effectively provide temporary relief.

Lifestyle Adjustments: Addressing contributing factors, such as ergonomics at work or stress management, can help prevent recurring muscle pain.

Professional Care: In cases of severe or chronic muscle pain, consultation with a healthcare provider, physical therapist, or chiropractor may be necessary to determine the underlying cause and receive appropriate treatment.

Natural remedies, including Arnica and Cayenne Pepper, can be part of a comprehensive approach to managing muscle pain.

Nausea and Vomiting

Nausea and Vomiting: Causes and Management: Nausea and vomiting are common symptoms that can arise from various underlying causes. These symptoms can be quite uncomfortable and may occur due to factors such as

Gastrointestinal Infections: Viral or bacterial infections of the stomach and intestines can lead to nausea and vomiting.

Motion Sickness: Motion-related activities, such as car rides, boat trips, or amusement park rides, can trigger motion sickness and its associated symptoms.

Pregnancy: Morning sickness is common during pregnancy, often characterized by nausea and vomiting.

Medications: Certain medications can induce nausea and vomiting as side effects. Chemotherapy drugs are one example.

Migraines: Severe headaches, known as migraines, can accompany nausea and vomiting.

Food Poisoning: Consuming contaminated food or beverages can result in gastrointestinal distress.

Management and relief from nausea and vomiting often involve several strategies, depending on the cause and severity.

Dietary Modifications: Eating bland, easily digestible foods and staying hydrated can help manage nausea and prevent dehydration. Ginger, crackers, and clear liquids are often recommended.

Hydration: Staying well-hydrated is crucial, especially if vomiting is frequent. Sipping water, clear broths, or electrolyte beverages can help maintain fluid balance.

Rest: Adequate rest can assist in the recovery process and alleviate symptoms.

Medications: Over the counter or prescription antiemetic medications can effectively manage nausea and vomiting. These medications work by reducing nausea and preventing vomiting.

Avoiding Triggers: If you know specific triggers, such as certain foods or odors, it is advisable to avoid them.

Acupressure Bands: Wristbands designed to stimulate acupressure points may help alleviate nausea and vomiting for some individuals.

Ginger (Zingiber officinale): Ginger is a natural remedy known for its anti-nausea properties. Ginger candies, ginger tea, or ginger supplements can be effective.

Mint and Peppermint (Mentha × piperita): Mint and peppermint may help relieve nausea. Peppermint candies, tea, or inhalation of mint aroma can be soothing.

Prescription Medications: Healthcare providers may prescribe stronger medications for symptom relief in severe or persistent cases.

It is important to address nausea and vomiting promptly, as they can lead to dehydration and malnutrition if left unmanaged. If symptoms persist, become severe, or are associated with other concerning signs, it is advisable to consult a healthcare provider for a thorough evaluation and personalized treatment plan.

Osteoarthritis

Osteoarthritis is a common joint condition characterized by the deterioration of cartilage, leading to pain, stiffness, and reduced mobility. In addition to conventional treatments, individuals with osteoarthritis often explore natural supplements like Turmeric (Curcuma longa) and Boswellia (Boswellia serrata) to help manage their symptoms.

Causes:

Age: Osteoarthritis is more prevalent with age, as joint wear and tear accumulate over time.

Joint Injury: Previous joint injuries or surgeries can increase the risk of osteoarthritis in affected joints.

Genetics: Family history and genetic factors may contribute to the development of osteoarthritis.

Obesity: Excess body weight increases stress on weight-bearing joints, increasing the risk of osteoarthritis.

Joint Overuse: Repetitive use or activities that stress the joints can lead to cartilage damage.

Joint Pain: Osteoarthritis typically results in joint pain that worsens with movement and improves with rest.

Stiffness: Affected joints can become stiff, particularly after periods of inactivity.

Reduced Range of Motion: Osteoarthritis can limit the range of motion in the affected joint.

Grating Sensation: Some individuals may experience a grating or crackling sensation when moving the joint.

Joint Enlargement: In advanced cases, the joint may appear enlarged due to the formation of bony outgrowth.

Turmeric (Curcuma longa): Curcumin, the active compound in turmeric, is known for its anti-inflammatory and antioxidant properties. Turmeric supplements or adding turmeric to your diet may help reduce inflammation and alleviate osteoarthritis-related pain. Consult with a healthcare provider for appropriate dosages and safety.

Boswellia (Boswellia serrata): Boswellia, or Indian frankincense, contains compounds that have anti-inflammatory and analgesic effects. Boswellia supplements can help reduce pain and improve joint function.

Traditional Management:

Pain Relief: Over-the-counter pain relievers like acetaminophen or nonsteroidal anti-inflammatory drugs (NSAIDs) can help manage pain.

Lifestyle Modifications: Maintaining a healthy weight, engaging in low-impact exercises, and protecting joints during daily activities are crucial.

Physical Therapy: Physical therapy can enhance joint function and guide exercises and stretches.

Assistive Devices: Braces, splints, or canes can offer joint support and alleviate pain.

Topical Creams: Topical creams with capsaicin or NSAIDs can be applied directly to the affected joint for pain relief.

Injections: Corticosteroid or hyaluronic acid injections can temporarily relieve pain when administered directly into the joint.

Surgery: In severe cases, joint replacement surgery may be considered to replace the damaged joint with an artificial one.

Alternative Therapies: Some individuals explore alternative treatments like acupuncture, acupuncture, or supplements such as glucosamine and chondroitin. It is important to discuss these options with a healthcare provider.

Osteoporosis

Osteoporosis, a condition characterized by bone density loss and increased fracture risk, can be managed, and even prevented through various strategies, including natural remedies such as Horsetail (Equisetum arvense), Red Clover (Trifolium pratense), and other effective approaches:

Causes and Risk Factors:

Aging: Osteoporosis risk rises with age, especially after menopause in women.

Hormonal Changes: Decreased estrogen levels in menopause and low testosterone in men can contribute to bone loss.

Family History: A family history of osteoporosis or fractures may elevate risk.

Low Body Weight: Being underweight or having a small frame can increase susceptibility.

Diet and Nutrition: Adequate calcium and vitamin D intake is crucial for strong bones. Include dairy, leafy greens, and fortified foods in your diet. Supplements may be recommended.

Physical Activity: Weight-bearing exercises, like walking and resistance training, can enhance bone density. Balance exercises reduce fall risks.

Lifestyle Choices: Smoking and excessive alcohol consumption weaken bones and should be avoided.

Medical Conditions: Certain diseases and medications may elevate the risk of osteoporosis.

Symptoms: Osteoporosis is often asymptomatic until a fracture occurs, leading to hip, vertebral, and wrist fractures.

Natural Remedies and Management:

Horsetail (Equisetum arvense): Horsetail is rich in silica, a mineral that supports bone health. It can be consumed as an herbal tea or taken as a supplement. Consult a healthcare provider for proper dosages.

Red Clover (Trifolium pratense): Red clover contains compounds that may help maintain bone density. It is available as a dietary supplement or in tea form.

Calcium and Vitamin D: A diet rich in calcium and vitamin D is essential. Dairy products, leafy greens, fortified foods, and supplements can help meet these requirements.

Regular Exercise: Weight-bearing exercises, balance training, and strength exercises can improve bone density and overall health.

Medications:
In cases of severe osteoporosis, a healthcare provider may prescribe bisphosphonates, hormone therapy, or other medications to slow bone loss and reduce fracture risk.

Fall Prevention: Minimizing fall risks through home modifications and assistive devices is vital.

Lifestyle Choices: Quit smoking and limit alcohol consumption for bone health.

Bone Density Testing: Regular bone density scans help assess bone health and treatment needs.

Osteoporosis management and prevention strategies should be personalized based on individual risk factors and health status. Consultation with a healthcare provider, particularly for those at higher risk, can lead to a tailored plan for maintaining strong bones and reducing fracture risks.

Pain and Inflammation

Pain and inflammation are common responses to various health conditions and injuries. Understanding their causes and strategies for management is essential for overall well-being. In addition to conventional approaches, natural remedies such as White Willow (Salix alba), Turmeric (Curcuma longa), and Devil's Claw (Harpagophytum procumbens) can complement pain and inflammation management.

Causes:

Injury: Acute sprains, strains, or fractures often result in localized pain and inflammation.

Infections: Inflammatory responses are common when the body combats infections, whether bacterial, viral, or fungal.

Chronic Conditions: Conditions such as arthritis, autoimmune diseases, and certain cancers can lead to persistent pain and inflammation.

Overuse: Repetitive movements and overuse of specific body parts can result in localized inflammation and pain.

Diet and Lifestyle: Poor dietary choices, excessive alcohol consumption, and smoking can contribute to chronic inflammation and pain.

Management Strategies:

Rest and Immobilization: Rest and immobilization of the affected area for acute injuries can reduce pain and inflammation.

Cold and Heat Therapy: Applying ice can reduce swelling, while heat can alleviate muscle tension and promote blood flow.

Medications:
Non-prescription pain relievers (NSAIDs) like ibuprofen relieve pain and reduce inflammation. Prescription medications may be necessary for more severe conditions.

Physical Therapy: Rehabilitation exercises and therapies can improve mobility, reduce pain, and enhance muscle strength.

Diet and Nutrition: Consuming an anti-inflammatory diet rich in fruits, vegetables, and omega-3 fatty acids can help manage chronic inflammation.

Lifestyle Changes: Quitting smoking and moderating alcohol consumption can reduce inflammation.

Supplements:
Some supplements like turmeric, devil's claw, and white willow have anti-inflammatory properties and can complement pain management.

Acupuncture and Acupressure: These alternative therapies can provide pain relief for some individuals.

Mind-Body Techniques: Meditation, yoga, and relaxation techniques can help manage chronic pain and inflammation.

Prescription Medications: Sometimes, healthcare providers may prescribe stronger medications to manage pain and inflammation, especially for chronic conditions.

Surgery: Surgical interventions may be necessary for severe injuries or conditions that do not respond to other treatments.

Pain and inflammation are common responses to various health conditions and injuries. Understanding their causes and strategies for management is essential for overall well-being. In addition to conventional approaches, natural supplements can provide valuable support in managing pain and inflammation. Here, we explore some of these supplements individually:

White Willow (Salix alba): White Willow bark contains salicin, a compound similar to aspirin. It has anti-inflammatory and pain-relieving properties. This supplement can be taken in various forms, such as capsules, teas, or liquid extracts, under the guidance of a healthcare provider.

Turmeric (Curcuma longa): Turmeric contains curcumin, a powerful anti-inflammatory and antioxidant compound. Curcumin supplements are available and can help alleviate pain and inflammation. Curcumin absorption can be enhanced when taken with black pepper.

Devil's Claw (Harpagophytum procumbens): Devil's Claw is known for its anti-inflammatory properties. It may help reduce pain in conditions like osteoarthritis. Devil's Claw supplements come in various forms, and a healthcare provider should determine the recommended dosage.

These natural supplements can be a valuable addition to pain and inflammation management, but it is crucial to use them under the guidance of a healthcare provider. The effectiveness of these supplements may vary from person to person, and their use should be tailored to individual needs and health conditions. Maintaining a healthy lifestyle, including a balanced diet and regular physical activity, is important for overall well-being and reducing the risk of chronic inflammation.

Pain Management

Pain is a common experience and can result from various causes. Effective pain management involves understanding the underlying causes and employing various strategies to alleviate discomfort. Here, we explore the causes of pain and comprehensive strategies for its management.

Causes:

Injury: Acute sprains, strains, and fractures often lead to localized pain.

Medical Conditions: Chronic conditions such as arthritis, fibromyalgia, and cancer can cause persistent pain.

Inflammation: Inflammatory responses to infections or chronic inflammation can result in pain.

Neuropathy: Nerve damage from conditions like diabetes can lead to neuropathic pain.

Overuse: Repetitive movements and overuse of specific body parts can result in localized pain.

Comprehensive Pain Management Strategies:

Medications: Non-prescription pain relievers (e.g., NSAIDs) or prescription medications relieve pain. Opioid medications should be used with caution and under healthcare provider guidance.

Physical Therapy: Rehabilitation exercises and therapies improve mobility, reduce pain, and enhance muscle strength.

Interventional Procedures: Nerve blocks or epidural injections can relieve pain for specific pain conditions.

Psychological Support: Counseling and cognitive-behavioral therapy can help individuals cope with chronic pain.

Complementary and Alternative Therapies: Techniques such as acupuncture, acupressure, and chiropractic care can relieve some individuals.

Lifestyle Changes: Maintaining a balanced diet, regular exercise, and managing stress can reduce the risk of chronic pain.

Pain-Relieving Creams and Gels: Topical products containing substances like capsaicin or NSAIDs can be applied directly to the affected area.

Assistive Devices: Braces, splints, or orthotics can support and alleviate pain in affected areas.

Mind-Body Techniques: Meditation, yoga, and relaxation techniques can help manage chronic pain.

Surgery: In severe cases or when other methods are ineffective, surgical procedures may be considered.

Natural Supplements: Natural supplements like turmeric, white willow, and devil's claw have anti-inflammatory properties and can complement pain management. A healthcare provider should guide their use.

Turmeric (Curcuma longa): Turmeric is famed for its active compound, curcumin, which exhibits potent anti-inflammatory and antioxidant properties. It is particularly effective in managing pain associated with inflammatory conditions such as arthritis. Turmeric supplements are available, and a healthcare provider can recommend their daily dosage. Combining turmeric with black pepper can enhance curcumin absorption.

White Willow (Salix alba): White Willow bark contains salicin, a compound akin to aspirin. It possesses anti-inflammatory and pain-relieving attributes. This supplement is available in various forms, including capsules, teas, and liquid extracts, and should be used following the guidance of a healthcare provider.

Devil's Claw (Harpagophytum procumbens): Devil's Claw is renowned for its anti-inflammatory properties. It has demonstrated efficacy in reducing pain associated with conditions like osteoarthritis. Devil's Claw supplements come in diverse forms, and it is prudent to establish the appropriate dosage with the assistance of a healthcare provider.

These natural supplements can be valuable components of a comprehensive pain management strategy. It is essential to underscore the importance of consulting with a healthcare provider before integrating them into one's pain management regimen. The effectiveness of these supplements can vary among individuals, and their utilization should be tailored to individual needs and health conditions. Additionally, maintaining a healthy lifestyle, which encompasses a balanced diet and regular physical activity, plays a pivotal role in overall well-being and the mitigation of chronic pain.

Parkinson's Disease

Parkinson's Disease is a complex neurodegenerative condition that affects movement and can cause a range of symptoms. While there is no cure for Parkinson's Disease, certain natural supplements, including Coenzyme Q10 (CoQ10) and Turmeric (Curcuma longa), have shown promise in providing supportive strategies.

Causes:

Neurodegeneration: Parkinson's Disease is primarily caused by the gradual loss of dopamine-producing cells in the brain. Genetics: Some cases of Parkinson's Disease have a genetic component, where specific gene mutations increase the risk.

Environmental Factors: Exposure to certain toxins, such as pesticides, has been associated with an increased risk of Parkinson's Disease.

Comprehensive Management Strategies:

Medications: Healthcare providers may prescribe medications that help manage the symptoms of Parkinson's Disease, such as levodopa and dopamine agonists.

Physical and Occupational Therapy: Physical and occupational therapists can assist in managing mobility and daily living challenges.

Exercise: Regular physical activity can improve mobility, balance, and overall well-being for individuals with Parkinson's Disease.

Diet: A balanced diet rich in fruits, vegetables, and whole grains can help maintain general health.

Supplements: Certain supplements may provide supportive benefits.

Coenzyme Q10 (CoQ10): CoQ10 is an antioxidant that may help improve cell energy production. Research suggests it may have a neuroprotective effect in Parkinson's Disease.

Turmeric (Curcuma longa): The active compound in turmeric, curcumin, has anti-inflammatory and antioxidant properties that may be beneficial in managing inflammation associated with Parkinson's Disease.

Deep Brain Stimulation (DBS): In some cases, DBS surgery may be recommended to alleviate symptoms.

It is important to note that while supplements like CoQ10 and turmeric have shown potential benefits, they should be used under the guidance of a healthcare provider and should not replace prescribed medications or other essential aspects of treatment. Parkinson's Disease management is personalized, and a healthcare provider can tailor a plan to meet individual needs and preferences.

Post-Traumatic Stress Disorder (PTSD)

Post-Traumatic Stress Disorder (PTSD) is a mental health condition that can develop after experiencing a traumatic event. Effective management involves understanding its causes and employing strategies to alleviate symptoms.

Causes:

Trauma: PTSD often arises after experiencing or witnessing a traumatic event, such as combat, assault, accidents, or natural disasters.

Biological Factors: Individual differences in brain structure and function can contribute to the development of PTSD.

Psychological Factors: Coping strategies, personality traits, and previous life experiences can influence one's risk of developing PTSD.

Comprehensive Management Strategies:

Psychotherapy: Cognitive-behavioral therapy (CBT), exposure therapy, and eye movement desensitization and reprocessing (EMDR) are effective forms of psychotherapy for managing PTSD.

Medications: Antidepressants like selective serotonin reuptake inhibitors (SSRIs) can help manage symptoms, including anxiety and depression.

Supportive Interventions: Supportive therapies, group counseling, and family therapy can assist individuals in managing the emotional impact of PTSD.

Lifestyle and Self-Care: Regular physical activity, a balanced diet, and good sleep hygiene can improve overall well-being.

Mindfulness and Relaxation Techniques: Mindfulness meditation, yoga, and relaxation exercises can help manage symptoms and improve emotional regulation.

Avoidance of Triggers: Individuals with PTSD are encouraged to avoid situations and triggers that exacerbate symptoms.

Medication for Specific Symptoms: In some cases, medications may be prescribed to manage specific symptoms, such as nightmares or insomnia.

Service Animals: Service dogs can provide emotional support and assistance to individuals with PTSD.

Natural Supplements: Some natural supplements like melatonin and ashwagandha may help alleviate symptoms and support overall well-being.

Ashwagandha (Withania somnifera): Ashwagandha is an adaptogenic herb that may help reduce stress and anxiety. It is available in supplement form and should be used under the guidance of a healthcare provider.

Melatonin: Melatonin is a hormone that regulates sleep-wake cycles. Some individuals with PTSD may experience sleep disturbances, and melatonin supplements can help improve sleep quality. A healthcare provider can recommend appropriate dosages.

Effective management of PTSD often involves a combination of these strategies tailored to individual needs. Working closely with mental health professionals, including therapists and psychiatrists, is essential for developing a personalized plan that addresses the unique aspects of one's PTSD and provides the best possible quality of life.

Premenstrual Syndrome (PMS)

Premenstrual Syndrome (PMS) is a common condition characterized by a range of physical and emotional symptoms that occur in the days leading up to menstruation. In addition to conventional management strategies, herbal remedies can offer a complementary approach to alleviating PMS symptoms. Here, we delve into some herbal remedies individually, exploring their potential roles in managing PMS:

Chasteberry (Vitex agnus-castus): Chasteberry, also known as Vitex, is an herbal remedy that has gained popularity for its potential to alleviate PMS symptoms. It is believed to influence hormonal balance, by affecting the pituitary gland and normalizing the menstrual cycle. Chasteberry supplements are available and can be a part of a comprehensive PMS management plan. The recommended dosage should be determined with the guidance of a healthcare provider.

Dong Quai (Angelica sinensis): Dong Quai is a traditional Chinese herb used for centuries to address women's health concerns, including PMS symptoms. It is believed to help regulate hormonal fluctuations and reduce menstrual pain. Dong Quai supplements are available and should be discussed with a healthcare provider to determine the appropriate dosage.

Black Cohosh (Actaea racemosa): Black Cohosh is an herbal remedy with a history of use in addressing various women's health issues, including menopausal symptoms. Some individuals find it helpful in managing PMS symptoms, particularly mood-related ones. Black Cohosh supplements can be considered with the guidance of a healthcare provider.

Evening Primrose Oil (Oenothera biennis): Evening Primrose Oil is a source of gamma-linolenic acid (GLA) source. This essential fatty acid may help reduce breast tenderness and mood swings associated with PMS. It is available in supplement form, and its use and dosage should be discussed with a healthcare provider.

It is important to note that herbal remedies can vary in effectiveness among individuals, and a healthcare provider should guide their use. These remedies should complement, not replace, conventional management strategies, such as lifestyle modifications, medications, and counseling. An individualized approach to PMS management is essential, and healthcare providers can tailor a plan to meet specific needs and preferences. Regular check-ups and adjustments to the management plan may be necessary to ensure the best possible quality of life during the premenstrual phase.

Prostate Disorders

Prostate disorders affect the prostate gland, a small, walnut-shaped organ in men that produces seminal fluid. Effective management involves understanding the causes and employing strategies to address specific disorders, such as benign prostatic hyperplasia (BPH) or prostate cancer.

Causes: Benign Prostatic Hyperplasia (BPH): BPH is often attributed to age-related changes in the prostate, causing the gland to enlarge and potentially obstruct the urethra.

Prostatitis: Prostatitis is typically caused by a bacterial infection or inflammation of the prostate gland.

Prostate Cancer: The exact causes of prostate cancer are not fully understood, but it is believed to result from genetic and environmental factors.

Comprehensive Management Strategies:

Medications: Alpha-blockers and 5-alpha reductase inhibitors can help relax the prostate and reduce its size.

Minimally Invasive Procedures: Transurethral microwave therapy (TUMT) and transurethral needle ablation (TUNA) can alleviate BPH symptoms.

Surgery: In more severe cases, surgical procedures like transurethral resection of the prostate (TURP) may be recommended.

Antibiotics: Bacterial prostatitis is treated with antibiotics to eliminate the infection.

Pain Medication: Nonsteroidal anti-inflammatory drugs (NSAIDs) can help alleviate pain and inflammation.

Alpha-Blockers: These medications may relax the prostate and bladder neck muscles, reducing discomfort.

Prostate Cancer:

Treatment Options: The management of prostate cancer depends on the stage and aggressiveness of the cancer. Options include active surveillance, surgery, radiation therapy, hormone therapy, chemotherapy, and immunotherapy.

Diet and Lifestyle: A diet rich in fruits, vegetables, and whole grains can support prostate health. Regular exercise and maintaining a healthy weight are associated with a reduced risk of prostate disorders.

Herbal Remedies: Prostate disorders, including benign prostatic hyperplasia (BPH) and prostatitis, can bring about bothersome symptoms that affect a man's quality of life. In addition to conventional treatment options, some herbal remedies have shown potential in addressing these disorders. Here, we delve into two herbal remedies individually, exploring their roles in managing prostate health:

Saw Palmetto (Serenoa repens): Saw Palmetto is derived from the fruit of the saw palmetto plant and has been studied for its potential benefits in managing BPH, a condition characterized by the non-cancerous enlargement of the prostate gland. Saw Palmetto is believed to work by inhibiting the action of the hormone dihydrotestosterone (DHT) on prostate tissue, reducing inflammation, and promoting healthy prostate function. It is available in various forms, including supplements, and should be used under the guidance of a healthcare provider to determine the appropriate dosage.

Pygeum (Prunus africana): Pygeum is an herbal remedy extracted from the bark of the African plum tree. It has been explored for its potential to alleviate BPH symptoms, particularly those related to urinary function. Pygeum is believed to have anti-inflammatory and anti-androgenic properties. It is available as a supplement, and its use and dosage should be discussed with a healthcare provider.

It is important to emphasize that herbal remedies should complement, not replace, conventional medical treatments. While some individuals may find relief from herbal supplements like Saw Palmetto and Pygeum, their effectiveness can vary among individuals. Collaborating closely with a healthcare provider is essential to ensure that these remedies are integrated safely and effectively into the overall management plan for prostate disorders. Regular check-ins and adjustments to the management plan may be necessary to optimize prostate health and overall well-being.

Living with a prostate disorder can have emotional and psychological implications. Counseling and support groups can provide emotional support and strategies for coping.

Effective management of prostate disorders often involves a combination of these strategies tailored to the specific condition and individual needs. Healthcare providers play a critical role in developing a personalized plan that addresses the unique aspects of each disorder and provides the best possible quality of life. Regular check-ups and discussions with healthcare providers are essential for monitoring and adjusting the management plan.

Psoriasis

Psoriasis is a chronic skin condition characterized by the rapid growth of skin cells, leading to the formation of red, itchy, and scaly patches on the skin. Effective management involves understanding its causes and employing various strategies to alleviate symptoms and maintain skin health.

Causes:

Genetics: Psoriasis tends to run in families, suggesting a genetic predisposition.

Immune System Dysfunction: An overactive immune system can trigger the rapid growth of skin cells.

Environmental Factors: Psoriasis symptoms may be exacerbated by environmental factors such as stress, infections, and injury to the skin.

Comprehensive Management Strategies:

Topical Treatments:

Corticosteroids: These anti-inflammatory creams or ointments can help reduce redness and itching.

Topical Retinoids: These medications help slow down the growth of skin cells and reduce inflammation.

Coal Tar Products: Shampoos, creams, and bath solutions containing coal tar can alleviate symptoms.

Salicylic Acid: This can help promote the shedding of dead skin cells and reduce scaling.

Phototherapy: Ultraviolet (UV) Light: Controlled exposure to UVB or UVA light can slow down skin cell growth and alleviate symptoms.

Oral and Injectable Medications:

Lifestyle and Self-Care:

Moisturizers: Regular use of moisturizers can help reduce dryness and itching.

Stress Management: Stress reduction techniques such as meditation and relaxation can help alleviate symptoms.

Avoiding Triggers: Identifying and avoiding triggers that worsen psoriasis, such as certain medications or skin injuries.

Herbal Remedies:

In addition to conventional treatments, herbal remedies can offer a complementary approach to alleviate symptoms and support overall skin health. Here, we delve into some herbal remedies individually, exploring their potential roles in managing psoriasis:

Aloe Vera (Aloe barbadensis miller): Aloe vera is a succulent plant known for its soothing and moisturizing properties. When applied topically, aloe vera gel can help reduce redness, itching, and inflammation associated with psoriasis plaques. Its natural cooling effect provides relief, making it a popular choice among individuals with psoriasis. Pure aloe vera gel can be applied directly to affected areas of the skin. Some individuals may prefer to use commercially available aloe vera gels or lotions.

Oregon Grape (Mahonia aquifolium): Oregon grape is an herbal remedy that contains berberine, a compound with anti-inflammatory and antimicrobial properties. Some find creams or ointments containing Oregon grape extract can alleviate psoriasis symptoms, particularly when applied topically. The ointments can be applied to affected areas as directed on the product label or as a healthcare provider recommends.

It is important to note that herbal remedies vary in effectiveness among individuals, and a healthcare provider should guide their use. These remedies should complement, not replace, conventional treatments and skincare routines. Collaborating closely with a healthcare provider is essential to ensure that these remedies are integrated safely and effectively into the overall management plan for psoriasis. Regular check-ins and adjustments to the management plan may be necessary to optimize skin health and overall well-being.

Effective management of psoriasis often involves a combination of these strategies tailored to individual needs. Regular check-ups and discussions with healthcare providers are essential to monitor and adjust the management plan to maintain skin health and overall well-being.

Respiratory Conditions

Respiratory conditions encompass various health issues affecting the lungs and the airways. Effective management involves understanding the causes and employing various strategies to alleviate symptoms and improve lung health.

Causes:

Infections: Bacterial, viral, and fungal infections can lead to respiratory conditions such as pneumonia, bronchitis, and tuberculosis.

Environmental Factors: Exposure to pollutants, allergens, and irritants can contribute to respiratory conditions, including asthma and chronic obstructive pulmonary disease (COPD).

Genetics: Conditions like cystic fibrosis have a genetic component.

Comprehensive Management Strategies:

Medications:

Bronchodilators: These medications relax the airway muscles, making breathing easier.

Corticosteroids: These anti-inflammatory drugs can reduce airway inflammation.

Antibiotics: Prescribed to treat respiratory infections caused by bacteria.

Lifestyle Modifications:

Quitting Smoking: Smoking cessation is critical for individuals with respiratory conditions to prevent further damage.

Environmental Control: Reducing exposure to allergens and irritants, such as dust mites, pollen, and air pollutants.

Regular Exercise: Physical activity can improve lung function and overall respiratory health.

Oxygen Therapy: Supplemental oxygen may be prescribed for individuals with severe respiratory conditions to ensure adequate oxygen levels in the blood.

Pulmonary Rehabilitation: Comprehensive programs that include exercise, education, and emotional support to help individuals manage their condition.

Respiratory conditions can be challenging, but herbal remedies offer an alternative approach to support lung health and alleviate symptoms associated with asthma and chronic obstructive pulmonary disease (COPD). Here, we explore some herbal remedies individually, shedding light on their potential roles in respiratory health:

Eucalyptus (Eucalyptus globulus): Eucalyptus is known for its ability to ease respiratory symptoms. Its active compound, cineole, is believed to have anti-inflammatory and decongestant properties. Eucalyptus oil can be used in steam inhalation, which involves adding a few drops to hot water and inhaling the steam. This can help open airways and relieve congestion.

Ginger (Zingiber officinale): Ginger is a versatile herb known for its anti-inflammatory and antioxidant properties. Some individuals find ginger can help ease respiratory symptoms by reducing inflammation and improving airflow. It can be consumed as ginger tea, added to meals, or used in an infusion.

Peppermint (Mentha × piperita): Peppermint contains menthol, a natural decongestant. Peppermint tea or steam inhalation with peppermint oil can relieve respiratory symptoms, particularly congestion and throat irritation.

It is important to emphasize that herbal remedies should complement, not replace, conventional medical treatments and therapies. The effectiveness of herbal remedies may vary among individuals, and a healthcare provider should guide their use. Collaborating closely with a healthcare provider ensures that these remedies are integrated safely and effectively into the overall management plan for respiratory conditions. Regular check-ins and adjustments to the management plan may be necessary to optimize lung health and overall well-being.

Respiratory therapists can teach techniques such as breathing exercises and inhalers. Effective management of respiratory conditions often involves a combination of these strategies tailored to the specific condition and individual needs.

Rheumatoid Arthritis

Rheumatoid arthritis (RA) is a chronic autoimmune condition that primarily affects the joints, leading to inflammation, pain, and potential joint damage. Effective management involves understanding the causes and employing various strategies to alleviate symptoms and preserve joint health.

Causes:

Autoimmune Response: Rheumatoid arthritis is triggered by an abnormal immune system response. The immune system mistakenly attacks the synovium, the lining of the membranes that surround the joints.

Genetic Factors: RA has a genetic component, and a family history of the condition can increase one's risk.

Environmental Factors: Factors such as smoking, exposure to certain pollutants, and infections may contribute to the development of RA.

Comprehensive Management Strategies:

Medications:

Disease-Modifying Antirheumatic Drugs (DMARDs): These medications slow the progression of RA by suppressing the overactive immune response.

Nonsteroidal Anti-Inflammatory Drugs (NSAIDs): NSAIDs can help manage pain and inflammation.

Biologics: Biologic drugs target specific parts of the immune system to reduce inflammation.

Lifestyle Modifications:

Physical Activity: Regular exercise can help maintain joint flexibility and overall health.

Dietary Changes: Some individuals find relief from RA symptoms by making dietary adjustments, such as consuming anti-inflammatory   foods.
Weight Management: Maintaining a healthy weight can reduce stress on joints.

Physical and Occupational Therapy: These therapies can help individuals learn how to protect their joints and improve their overall quality of life.

Herbal Remedies:

Rheumatoid arthritis (RA) is an autoimmune disorder that affects the joints, causing pain, inflammation, and stiffness. In addition to conventional treatments, some herbal remedies have shown promise in managing RA symptoms and supporting joint health. Here, we explore two herbal remedies individually, highlighting their potential roles in managing RA:

Turmeric (Curcuma longa): Turmeric is well-known for its active compound, curcumin, which possesses anti-inflammatory and antioxidant properties. Some individuals with RA find that turmeric supplementation can help reduce joint pain and inflammation. Curcumin's potential to modulate the immune system and combat inflammation is particularly interesting. Turmeric can be consumed as a spice in food, or turmeric supplements can be taken. The dosage and form of turmeric should be determined with the guidance of a healthcare provider.

Boswellia (Boswellia serrata): Boswellia, also known as Indian frankincense, is another herbal remedy with anti-inflammatory properties. It contains Boswellia acids, which may help reduce inflammation and alleviate joint pain. Some individuals find that boswellia supplements provide relief from RA symptoms. The appropriate dosage and form of boswellia should be discussed with a healthcare provider.

It is important to note that herbal remedies should be used with conventional medical treatments, not as substitutes. RA varies among individuals, and the effectiveness of herbal remedies can also differ. Collaboration with a healthcare provider is vital to ensure that these remedies are safely and effectively integrated into the overall management plan for RA. Regular check-ins and adjustments to the management plan may be necessary to optimize joint health and overall well-being.

Surgical options like joint replacement may be considered in cases of severe joint damage. Effective management of RA often involves a combination of these strategies tailored to the specific condition and individual needs. Collaboration with healthcare providers is essential to ensure the management plan is personalized and optimized to support joint health and overall well-being.

Schizophrenia

Schizophrenia is a complex mental health disorder that often requires a multifaceted approach to symptom management. In addition to conventional treatments, some individuals explore herbal remedies to complement their care plans. Here, we delve into some herbal remedies individually and comprehensive strategies for managing schizophrenia.

Herbal Remedies:

St. John's Wort (Hypericum perforatum): St. John's Wort is an herb known for its potential to alleviate symptoms of depression and anxiety. Some individuals with schizophrenia find that it can help improve mood and reduce feelings of hopelessness. It is available as a supplement, but its use should be discussed with a healthcare provider due to potential interactions with other medications.

Ginkgo Biloba (Ginkgo biloba): Ginkgo biloba is an herbal remedy with antioxidant properties that may enhance cognitive function and memory. Some individuals use it to address cognitive deficits associated with schizophrenia. The dosage and form of ginkgo biloba should be determined with the guidance of a healthcare provider.

Comprehensive Management Strategies:

Antipsychotic Medications: These are typically the cornerstone of schizophrenia treatment, addressing positive and negative symptoms.

Psychotherapy: Cognitive Behavioral Therapy (CBT) can help individuals manage distressing symptoms and improve their daily functioning.

Social Support: Engaging with supportive family and community networks can be instrumental in the recovery process.

Self-Help and Lifestyle Adjustments: Maintaining a structured routine, prioritizing physical health, and avoiding substance use are essential for self-help strategies.

Vocational and Social Skills Training: These programs can enhance an individual's ability to engage in work and social interactions.

It is crucial to note that herbal remedies in schizophrenia management should be discussed with a healthcare provider. Herbal supplements should complement, not replace, conventional treatments, and their effectiveness can vary among individuals. Collaboration with healthcare providers ensures these remedies are safely integrated into the overall management plan. Regular check-ins and adjustments to the management plan are necessary to optimize mental health and overall well-being.

Sinusitis

Sinusitis, characterized by inflammation of the sinuses, can be challenging to manage, but some individuals explore herbal remedies alongside conventional treatments for symptom relief and sinus health. Here, we delve into herbal remedies individually and comprehensive strategies for managing sinusitis.

Herbal Remedies:

Echinacea (Echinacea purpurea): Echinacea is known for its potential to boost the immune system and help the body fend off infections. Some individuals use Echinacea to reduce the severity and duration of sinusitis symptoms. Echinacea supplements can be taken, but their use should be discussed with a healthcare provider.

Ginger (Zingiber officinale): Ginger possesses anti-inflammatory and antimicrobial properties. It can help ease sinusitis symptoms and reduce inflammation in the nasal passages. Ginger can be consumed as ginger tea, added to meals, or used in an infusion.

Comprehensive Management Strategies:

Symptomatic Relief: Decongestants: Over the counter or prescription decongestants can temporarily relieve nasal congestion, though their use should be limited to a few days.

Saline Nasal Sprays: These sprays can help moisturize and clear the nasal passages.

Antibiotics:
In cases of acute bacterial sinusitis, antibiotics may be prescribed by a healthcare provider.

Nasal Corticosteroids: These medications can reduce inflammation and alleviate acute and chronic sinusitis symptoms.

Lifestyle Measures:

Steam Inhalation: Inhaling steam, infused with herbs like eucalyptus or chamomile, can ease congestion and relieve facial pain.

Hydration: Staying well-hydrated helps thin mucus and promote drainage.

Nasal Irrigation: Saline nasal irrigation, using a Neti pot or bulb syringe, can help remove mucus and irritants from the nasal passages.

Rest and Self-Care: Adequate rest and self-care measures, including avoiding irritants, can speed up recovery.

These remedies should complement conventional treatments, not replace them. Collaboration with healthcare providers ensures these remedies are safely and effectively integrated into the overall management plan. Regular check-ins and adjustments to the plan are necessary to optimize sinus health and overall well-being.

Skin Conditions

Skin conditions encompass a diverse array of disorders, and some individuals seek the benefits of herbal remedies to complement their management strategies. Here, we explore herbal remedies individually, along with comprehensive strategies for managing various skin conditions:

Herbal Remedies:

Aloe Vera (Aloe barbadensis miller): Aloe vera is renowned for its soothing properties and can benefit various skin conditions. Its cooling and anti-inflammatory effects make it a popular choice for burns, including sunburn. Apply aloe vera gel directly to the affected area for relief.

Chamomile (Matricaria chamomilla): Chamomile is known for its anti-inflammatory and calming properties. It can be beneficial for individuals with eczema. Chamomile tea can be used topically or as a compress to alleviate itching and inflammation.

Calendula (Calendula officinalis): Calendula possesses anti-inflammatory and antimicrobial properties. It is often used in creams, ointments, or oil infusions to soothe and heal irritated or damaged skin. It can be applied topically to the affected area.

Comprehensive Management Strategies:

Topical Treatments: Moisturizers: Keeping the skin well-hydrated is essential, especially for conditions like eczema and psoriasis.

Topical Corticosteroids: These effectively reduce inflammation and itching in many skin conditions.

Antifungal or Antibacterial Creams: These treat skin conditions caused by fungi or bacteria.

Medications:

Oral Medications: In some cases, oral medications like antihistamines or immunosuppressants may be prescribed.

Lifestyle Adjustments:

Dietary Changes: Identifying and avoiding trigger foods can help manage conditions like dermatitis herpetiformis.

Stress Management: Stress reduction techniques can be vital for managing stress-induced skin conditions.

Skin Protection: Sunscreen: Sun protection is crucial for various conditions and preventing skin cancer.

Avoiding Irritants: Identifying and avoiding skin irritants is essential for managing contact dermatitis and other sensitivities.

It is essential to consult with a healthcare provider before incorporating herbal remedies into the management plan for skin conditions, especially if you are taking other medications or have underlying health conditions. Herbal remedies should complement conventional treatments, not replace them.

Sleep Apnea

Sleep apnea is a sleep disorder characterized by repeated interruptions in breathing during sleep. Effective management involves understanding the causes and employing strategies to alleviate symptoms and improve sleep quality.

Causes:

Obstructive Sleep Apnea (OSA): This is the most typical form of sleep apnea and is typically caused by the relaxation of throat muscles, leading to airway obstruction during sleep.

Central Sleep Apnea: This type is less common and occurs when the brain fails to signal the muscles to breathe.

Complex Sleep Apnea Syndrome: Also known as treatment-emergent central sleep apnea, this is a combination of OSA and central sleep apnea.

Comprehensive Management Strategies:

Continuous Positive Airway Pressure (CPAP): A CPAP machine is the primary treatment for moderate to severe OSA. It delivers a constant stream of air to keep the airway open.

Bi-level Positive Airway Pressure (BiPAP): Like CPAP, BiPAP provides different pressure levels for inhalation and exhalation.

Oral Appliances: These devices, like mandibular advancement devices, reposition the jaw and tongue to keep the airway open.

Lifestyle Changes:

Weight Management: Losing excess weight can reduce the severity of sleep apnea, especially in cases where obesity is a contributing factor.

Positional Therapy: Sleeping on one's side can help prevent airway collapse in some individuals.

Herbal Remedies: While herbal remedies are not typically considered primary treatments for sleep apnea, some individuals explore them as complementary options to promote better sleep quality.

Valerian (Valeriana officinalis): Valerian is known for its calming and sedative properties. It may help individuals with mild sleep apnea relax and fall asleep more easily. Valerian is available in various forms, including capsules and herbal teas.

Lemon Balm (Melissa officinalis): Lemon balm is a soothing herb that can reduce anxiety and promote relaxation. It is often used in herbal teas and supplements to help improve sleep quality.

Passionflower (Passiflora incarnata): Passionflower is used for its calming effects and may benefit individuals with sleep apnea who have trouble falling asleep. It is available in various forms, including teas and supplements.

It is important to note that herbal remedies for sleep apnea should be discussed with a healthcare provider. These remedies should complement, not replace, conventional treatments.

Sleep Disorders

Sleep disorders encompass many conditions that affect an individual's ability to get restorative sleep. Effective management involves understanding the causes and employing strategies to alleviate symptoms and improve sleep quality.

Causes:

Insomnia: Often linked to stress, anxiety, or lifestyle factors, insomnia can make it difficult to fall or stay asleep.

Narcolepsy: This neurological disorder leads to excessive daytime sleepiness and sudden sleep attacks.

Restless Legs Syndrome (RLS): RLS is characterized by an uncontrollable urge to move the legs, often disrupting sleep.

Circadian Rhythm Disorders: Shift work, jet lag, and irregular sleep schedules can disrupt the body's internal clock.

Parasomnia: These disorders involve unusual behaviors during sleep, such as sleepwalking, night terrors, or sleep eating.

Comprehensive Management Strategies: Cognitive Behavioral Therapy for Insomnia (CBT-I): CBT-I is a structured program that helps individuals address the thoughts and behaviors contributing to insomnia.

Medications: Sometimes, healthcare providers may prescribe sleep medications or medications to address underlying causes.

Lifestyle Changes:

Sleep Hygiene: Establishing a consistent sleep routine, creating a comfortable sleep environment, and avoiding stimulants before bedtime can improve sleep quality.

Stress Management:

Techniques like relaxation exercises, meditation, or yoga can alleviate stress-related sleep issues.

Lifestyle Adjustments:

Weight Management: For conditions like sleep apnea, losing excess weight can significantly improve symptoms.

Dietary Changes: Avoiding heavy meals, caffeine, and alcohol close to bedtime can help individuals with sleep disorders.

Light Therapy: This is used for circadian rhythm disorders to help reset the body's internal clock, particularly in cases of jet lag or shift work.

Herbal Remedies: While herbal remedies are not typically considered primary treatments for sleep disorders, some individuals explore them as complementary options to promote better sleep quality.

Lavender (Lavandula angustifolia): Lavender is known for its calming and soothing effects. It can be used in aromatherapy, as an essential oil in a diffuser, or in herbal teas to improve sleep quality.

Chamomile (Matricaria chamomilla): Chamomile's anti-anxiety and sedative properties can make it a valuable option for addressing sleep disturbances. It is available as an herbal tea or in supplement form.

Valerian (Valeriana officinalis): Valerian's sedative effects can help individuals relax and fall asleep. Valerian is available in various forms, including capsules and herbal teas.

It is crucial to consult with a healthcare provider before incorporating herbal remedies into the management plan for sleep disorders. These remedies should complement, not replace, conventional treatments, and their effectiveness can vary among individuals. Collaboration with healthcare providers is vital to ensure these remedies are safely integrated into the overall management plan. Regular check-ins and adjustments to the plan are necessary to optimize sleep health and overall well-being.

Sore Throat

A sore throat, often characterized by pain, discomfort, and irritation, can result from various causes, such as infections or irritants. Effective management involves understanding the causes and employing strategies to alleviate symptoms and promote healing.

Causes:

Viral Infections: Many sore throats are caused by viruses, including the common cold or flu.

Bacterial Infections: Streptococcal bacteria can lead to strep throat, a bacterial infection causing a sore throat.

Environmental Factors: Exposure to irritants like smoke, pollutants, or dry air can lead to a sore throat.

Allergies: Allergic reactions can cause throat irritation and discomfort.

Comprehensive Management Strategies: Symptomatic Relief:

Pain Relievers: Over-the-counter pain relievers like acetaminophen or ibuprofen can help reduce pain and inflammation.

Throat Lozenges: Medicated lozenges or hard candies can temporarily relieve throat irritation.

Antibiotics: In cases of bacterial infections like strep throat, antibiotics may be prescribed by a healthcare provider.

Warm Saltwater Gargle: Gargling with warm salt water can soothe the throat and reduce inflammation.

Hydration: Staying well-hydrated with water, herbal teas, and warm soups can help keep the throat moist.

Humidification:
Using a humidifier can add moisture to the air and prevent throat dryness.

Herbal Remedies: Some herbal remedies are explored for their potential to alleviate sore throat symptoms.

Honey: Honey has natural antibacterial and soothing properties. It can be added to warm water or herbal tea. Please note that honey should not be given to infants under one year of age.

Sage (Salvia officinalis): Sage has anti-inflammatory and antimicrobial properties. It can be used in teas or gargled as a sage infusion.

Marshmallow Root (Althaea officinalis): Marshmallow root has a soothing effect and can help alleviate throat discomfort. It can be used to make teas or infusions.

It is important to consult with a healthcare provider before incorporating herbal remedies into the management plan for a sore throat, especially if you have underlying health conditions or are taking other medications. Herbal remedies should complement, not replace, conventional treatments. Collaboration with healthcare providers ensures these remedies are safely integrated into the overall management plan. Regular check-ins and adjustments to the plan are necessary to optimize throat health and overall well-being.

Stomach Ulcers

Stomach ulcers, also known as gastric ulcers or peptic ulcers, are open sores that develop on the inner lining of the stomach or the upper part of the small intestine. Effective management involves understanding the causes and employing strategies to alleviate symptoms and promote healing.

Causes:

Helicobacter pylori (H. pylori) Infection: This bacterium is a common cause of stomach ulcers.

Nonsteroidal Anti-Inflammatory Drugs (NSAIDs): Prolonged use of NSAIDs like aspirin or ibuprofen can lead to stomach ulcers.

Acid Production: Excessive stomach acid production can erode the stomach's protective lining and result in ulcers.

Comprehensive Management Strategies:

Medications:

Antibiotics: If H. pylori infection is detected, a healthcare provider may prescribe a combination of antibiotics to eradicate the bacterium.

Proton Pump Inhibitors (PPIs) and Histamine-2 (H2) Blockers: These medications reduce stomach acid production, allowing ulcers to heal.

Lifestyle Changes:

Avoiding NSAIDs: If possible, individuals with stomach ulcers should avoid or limit the use of NSAIDs.

Dietary Adjustments: Spicy foods, alcohol, and caffeine can exacerbate ulcer symptoms. A bland diet with small, frequent meals is often recommended.

Stress Management: High-stress levels can worsen ulcer symptoms. Stress reduction techniques like relaxation exercises or mindfulness can be beneficial.

Herbal Remedies: Some herbal remedies are explored to complement conventional ulcer management:

Licorice (Glycyrrhiza glabra):

Licorice root has been used in traditional medicine for its potential to soothe the stomach lining. DGL (deglycyrrhizinated licorice) is a form of licorice used for ulcers.

Aloe Vera (Aloe barbadensis miller): Aloe vera has anti-inflammatory and healing properties. It can be consumed as a juice or gel, but its use should be discussed with a healthcare provider.

Chamomile (Matricaria chamomilla): Chamomile tea may help alleviate indigestion and discomfort associated with ulcers.

It is important to consult with a healthcare provider before incorporating herbal remedies into the management plan for stomach ulcers, especially if you have underlying health conditions or are taking other medications. Herbal remedies should complement, not replace, conventional treatments. Collaboration with healthcare providers ensures that remedies are safely integrated into the management plan. Regular check-ins and adjustments to the plan are necessary to optimize ulcer healing and overall well-being.

Sunburn

Sunburn occurs when the skin is overexposed to ultraviolet (UV) radiation from the sun or artificial sources like tanning beds. Effective management involves understanding the causes and employing strategies to alleviate symptoms and promote healing. Causes:

UV Radiation: Exposure to UV radiation damages the DNA in skin cells and triggers an inflammatory response, leading to the characteristic redness and pain of sunburn.

Comprehensive Management Strategies:

Cool Compresses: Applying cool, damp compresses to sunburned areas can help alleviate heat and discomfort.

Pain Relievers: Over-the-counter pain relievers like ibuprofen can reduce pain and inflammation associated with sunburn.

Hydration: Drinking plenty of water can help maintain skin hydration and promote healing.

Moisturizers: A soothing, alcohol-free moisturizer, aloe vera gel, or hydrating cream can relieve dryness and discomfort.

Avoid Further Sun Exposure: Protect the sunburned area from further sun exposure until it heals. Wear protective clothing and apply sunscreen.

Herbal Remedies: Some herbal remedies are explored for their potential to alleviate sunburn symptoms and support skin healing.

Aloe Vera (Aloe barbadensis miller): Aloe vera gel is well-known for its cooling and soothing properties. Applying it directly to sunburned skin can help alleviate pain and redness.

Calendula (Calendula officinalis): Calendula cream or oil can be applied to the affected area to reduce inflammation and promote healing.

Lavender (Lavandula angustifolia) and Chamomile (Matricaria chamomilla): Lavender and chamomile essential oils can be diluted in a carrier oil and applied to sunburned skin. They have anti-inflammatory and soothing properties.

It is important to consult with a healthcare provider before incorporating herbal remedies into the management plan for sunburn, especially if you have underlying health conditions or are taking other medications. Herbal remedies should complement, not replace, conventional treatments. Collaboration with healthcare providers ensures these remedies are safely integrated into the overall management plan. Regular check-ins and adjustments to the plan are necessary to optimize sunburn healing and overall well-being.

Thyroid Disorders

Thyroid disorders encompass a range of conditions affecting the thyroid gland, which is crucial in regulating metabolism and other bodily functions. Effective management involves understanding the causes and employing strategies to alleviate symptoms and maintain thyroid health.

Causes:

Hypothyroidism occurs when the thyroid gland produces insufficient thyroid hormones. Autoimmune thyroiditis (Hashimoto's disease) is a common cause.

Hyperthyroidism: In hyperthyroidism, the thyroid gland overproduces thyroid hormones. Graves' disease is a frequent cause.

Comprehensive Management Strategies:

Medications:

Hypothyroidism: Replacement therapy with synthetic thyroid hormones (levothyroxine) is the primary treatment.

Hyperthyroidism: Medications like anti-thyroid drugs or beta-blockers may be prescribed to control hormone production.

Radioactive Iodine Treatment: Radioactive iodine may be used to reduce the activity of the thyroid gland in cases of hyperthyroidism.

Surgery: Surgical removal of the thyroid gland (thyroidectomy) is sometimes an option.

Lifestyle Changes:

Diet:
A diet rich in iodine and selenium is important for thyroid health.

Stress Management: Stress can exacerbate thyroid symptoms, so stress reduction techniques are beneficial.

Regular Monitoring: Periodic blood tests to measure thyroid hormone levels help adjust medication dosages and monitor the condition's progress.

Herbal Remedies: While herbal remedies are not typically considered primary treatments for thyroid disorders, some explore them as complementary options to support thyroid health.

Ashwagandha (Withania somnifera): Ashwagandha is an adaptogenic herb that may help regulate thyroid function and reduce stress.

Bladderwrack (Fucus vesiculosus): Bladderwrack is a seaweed containing iodine that may support thyroid health. It should be used under healthcare provider guidance due to iodine content.

Lemon Balm (Melissa officinalis): Lemon balm has calming properties and can help reduce stress, which is important for thyroid health.

It is essential to consult with a healthcare provider before incorporating herbal remedies into the management plan for thyroid disorders, especially if you have underlying health conditions or are taking other medications. Herbal remedies should complement, not replace, conventional treatments. Collaboration with healthcare providers ensures these remedies are safely integrated into the overall management plan. Regular check-ins and adjustments to the plan are necessary to optimize thyroid health and overall well-being.

Toothache

Toothache is a common dental issue characterized by pain or discomfort in or around a tooth. Effective management involves understanding the causes and employing strategies to alleviate symptoms and address underlying dental problems.

Causes:

Dental Decay (Cavities): Bacterial infections can lead to tooth decay, causing pain when the nerve inside the tooth is affected.

Gum Disease: Infections and inflammation of the gums can cause tooth pain, particularly when the roots of the teeth are exposed.

Tooth Fractures: Cracks or fractures in teeth can lead to toothache, especially when the nerve is exposed.

Impacted Wisdom Teeth: Wisdom teeth can become impacted, causing pain and discomfort.

Sinus Infections: Sometimes, pain in the upper teeth can be referred pain from sinus infections.

Comprehensive Management Strategies:

Dental Care:

Regular Dental Checkups: Routine dental visits can help identify and address dental issues before they become painful.

Treatment of Dental Problems: Dental professionals can provide treatments such as fillings, root canals, or extractions, as necessary.

Pain Management: Over-the-Counter Pain Relievers: Non-prescription pain relievers like acetaminophen or ibuprofen can help manage toothache pain.

Topical Anesthetics: Over-the-counter topical gels or ointments can temporarily numb the affected area.

Oral Hygiene: Proper Brushing and Flossing:

Maintaining good oral hygiene can prevent dental issues that lead to toothache.

Warm Saltwater Rinse: Gargling with warm salt water can help reduce inflammation and disinfect the affected area.

Herbal Remedies: Some herbal remedies are explored for their potential to alleviate toothache symptoms:

Clove (Syzygium aromaticum): Clove oil contains eugenol, a natural anesthetic. Applying a small amount to the affected area can temporarily numb the pain.

Peppermint (Mentha × piperita): Peppermint oil can be soothing and may be applied topically.

Guava Leaves (Psidium guajava): Chewing on guava leaves or using them to make mouthwash is a traditional remedy for toothache.

It is important to consult with a dental professional before incorporating herbal remedies into the management plan for toothache, especially if you have underlying dental issues. Herbal remedies should complement, not replace, conventional dental treatments. Collaboration with dental professionals ensures these remedies are safely integrated into the overall management plan. Regular dental checkups and adjustments to the plan are necessary to optimize oral health and overall well-being.

Urinary Tract Infections

Urinary tract infections are bacterial infections that affect any part of the urinary system, including the bladder, urethra, and kidneys. Effective management involves understanding the causes and employing strategies to alleviate symptoms and promote healing.

Causes:

Bacterial Infection: Most UTIs are caused by Escherichia coli (E. coli) bacteria, which enter the urinary system and multiply.

Comprehensive Management Strategies:

Antibiotics: UTIs are typically treated with a course of antibiotics prescribed by a healthcare provider. It is essential to complete the full course to clear the infection completely.

Hydration: Drinking plenty of water can help flush out bacteria from the urinary system and alleviate symptoms.

Cranberry Juice: Some studies suggest that cranberry juice may help prevent UTIs by inhibiting bacteria from sticking to the urinary tract.

Probiotics: Probiotic supplements containing beneficial bacteria can help maintain a healthy balance of microorganisms in the urinary and gastrointestinal tracts.

Herbal Remedies: While antibiotics are the primary treatment for UTIs, some individuals explore herbal remedies for their potential to complement conventional UTI management:

Dandelion (Taraxacum officinale): Dandelion leaf tea may act as a diuretic, promoting increased urine production and potentially helping flush out bacteria.

Goldenseal (Hydrastis canadensis): Goldenseal has antimicrobial properties and may be used as a natural remedy. However, it should be used under healthcare provider guidance.

Uva Ursi (Arctostaphylos uva-ursi): Uva ursi has been used traditionally for UTIs due to its antimicrobial properties. It should be used under healthcare provider guidance.

Viral Infections

Viral infections can affect various parts of the body, causing a wide range of illnesses. Effective management involves understanding the causes and strategies to alleviate symptoms and support the body's natural defense mechanisms.

Causes:

Viruses: Viral infections are caused by various viruses, including the common cold, influenza, herpes, and more.

Comprehensive Management Strategies:

Preventive Measures:

Vaccination: Vaccines can help prevent some viral infections, such as influenza, measles, and hepatitis.

Hand Hygiene: Regular handwashing with soap and water is essential to prevent the spread of viruses.

Avoiding Close Contact: During outbreaks, limiting close contact with infected individuals can reduce the risk of transmission.

Antiviral Medications: Some viral infections, like influenza or herpes, can be treated with antiviral medications prescribed by a healthcare provider.

Supportive Care: Rest, hydration, and a balanced diet can help the body's immune system fight viral infections.

Herbal Remedies: While antiviral medications are the primary treatment for many viral infections, some individuals explore herbal remedies for their potential to complement conventional viral infection management.

Echinacea (Echinacea purpurea): Echinacea stimulates the immune system and may be used as a natural remedy to support the body's defenses.

Astragalus (Astragalus membranaceus): Astragalus traditionally boosts the immune system's response to viral infections.

Lemon Balm (Melissa officinalis): Lemon balm may have antiviral properties and can be used in topical applications or tea.

It is important to consult with a healthcare provider before incorporating herbal remedies into the management plan for viral infections, especially if you have underlying health conditions or are taking other medications. Herbal remedies should complement, not replace, conventional treatments.

Weight Management

Weight management is a crucial aspect of overall health and well-being. Effective weight management involves understanding the causes of weight gain and employing strategies to achieve and maintain a healthy weight.

Causes:

Caloric Imbalance: Weight gain occurs when the number of calories consumed exceeds the number of calories burned through physical activity and metabolism.

Poor Diet: Consuming high-calorie, low-nutrient foods can contribute to weight gain.

Lack of Physical Activity: A sedentary lifestyle can lead to weight gain.

Genetics: Genetic factors can influence metabolism and how the body stores fat.

Comprehensive Management Strategies:

Balanced Diet: Caloric Control: Maintaining a balanced caloric intake is essential. Consult with a healthcare provider or nutritionist to determine an appropriate caloric goal.

Nutrient-rich foods: Focus on a diet rich in fruits, vegetables, lean proteins, and whole grains.

Portion Control: Be mindful of portion sizes to avoid overeating.

Regular Physical Activity: Regular exercise, such as walking, swimming, or strength training, can help burn calories and maintain a healthy weight.

Behavioral Changes: Identifying and addressing emotional or unhealthy eating habits can be essential for long-term weight management.

Support and Accountability: Consider seeking support from a healthcare provider, nutritionist, or a support group for weight management.

Stress Management: High-stress levels can lead to emotional eating. Stress reduction techniques like mindfulness, yoga, or meditation can be helpful.

Sleep: Aim for quality sleep, as poor sleep patterns can contribute to weight gain.

Herbal and Dietary Supplements: Some herbal and dietary supplements are explored for their potential to support weight management:

Garcinia Cambogia: Some studies suggest that garcinia cambogia may aid in weight loss by inhibiting fat production and reducing appetite.

Green Tea Extract: Green tea extract contains compounds that may increase metabolism and promote fat burning.

It is important to consult with a healthcare provider or a registered dietitian before incorporating herbal or dietary supplements into the weight management plan, especially if you have underlying health conditions. These supplements should complement, not replace, a balanced diet and regular exercise. Collaboration with healthcare providers ensures these remedies are safely integrated into the overall weight management plan. Regular check-ins and adjustments to the plan are necessary to achieve and maintain a healthy weight and overall well-being.

Wound Healing

Wound healing is a natural process that helps the body repair damaged tissue. Effective management involves understanding the causes of wounds and employing strategies to facilitate and optimize the healing process.

Causes:

Injury: Wounds can result from various forms of injury, including cuts, abrasions, burns, and surgical incisions.

Underlying Health Conditions: Certain health conditions, such as diabetes or vascular disease, can impair the body's ability to heal wounds.

Comprehensive Management Strategies:

Wound Care:

Cleaning: Gently clean the wound with mild soap and water to prevent infection.

Dressing: Applying an appropriate dressing can keep the wound clean and provide a moist environment conducive to healing.

Infection Prevention:

Antibiotics:
In cases of infected wounds, antibiotics may be prescribed by a healthcare provider.

Vaccinations:
Staying up to date with tetanus vaccinations is important, especially for puncture wounds.

Nutrition:
A diet rich in essential nutrients, particularly vitamin C, vitamin A, zinc, and protein, supports the healing process.

Hydration:
Staying well-hydrated is crucial for maintaining overall health, which, in turn, supports wound healing.

Rest and Stress Reduction: Adequate rest and stress reduction are essential for the body to direct its energy toward healing.

Herbal Remedies: Some herbal remedies are explored for their potential to facilitate wound healing and reduce inflammation:

Aloe Vera (Aloe barbadensis miller): Aloe vera gel can be applied topically to wounds to soothe and promote healing.

Calendula (Calendula officinalis): Calendula cream or oil may have anti-inflammatory and wound-healing properties.

Chamomile (Matricaria chamomilla): Chamomile essential oil or tea can have soothing and anti-inflammatory effects when applied to wounds.

It is essential to consult with a healthcare provider before incorporating herbal remedies into the wound healing process, especially if you have underlying health conditions or are taking other medications. Herbal remedies should complement, not replace, conventional wound care. Collaboration with healthcare providers ensures that these remedies are safely integrated into the wound-healing plan. Regular check-ins and adjustments to the plan are necessary to optimize wound healing and overall well-being.

Yeast Infections

Yeast infections are fungal infections caused by the overgrowth of Candida yeast. Effective management involves understanding the causes of yeast infections and employing strategies to alleviate symptoms and promote healing.

Causes:

Candida Overgrowth: Yeast infections are primarily caused by the overgrowth of Candida, a fungus that naturally resides in the body.

Antibiotic Use: Antibiotics can disrupt the balance of microorganisms in the body, potentially leading to yeast infections.

Weak Immune System: Conditions that weaken the immune system, such as diabetes or HIV, can make individuals more susceptible to yeast infections.

Comprehensive Management Strategies:

Antifungal Medications: Over-the-counter Treatments: ntifungal creams, ointments, and suppositories are available without a prescription for mild yeast infections.

Prescription Medications: Healthcare providers may prescribe oral antifungal medications for severe or recurring infections.

Lifestyle and Hygiene: Maintain Good Hygiene: Keep the genital area clean and dry, and avoid douching, which can disrupt the natural balance of microorganisms.

Wear Breathable Fabrics: Choose cotton underwear and avoid tight-fitting clothing.

Dietary Adjustments: Some individuals find that reducing sugar and refined carbohydrate intake can help prevent yeast infections.

Probiotics: Probiotic supplements containing beneficial bacteria can help maintain a healthy balance of microorganisms, including those that help control Candida.

Herbal Remedies: While antifungal medications are the primary treatment for yeast infections, some individuals explore herbal remedies for their potential to complement conventional management.

Tea Tree Oil (Melaleuca alternifolia): Tea tree oil has antifungal properties and can be diluted and applied topically to the affected area.

Garlic (Allium sativum): Garlic contains allicin, a compound with potential antifungal properties. Some individuals use garlic as a natural remedy by inserting a garlic clove into the vagina overnight.

Oregano Oil (Origanum vulgare): Oregano oil may have antifungal properties and can be diluted and applied topically.

It is crucial to consult with a healthcare provider before incorporating herbal remedies into the management plan for yeast infections, especially if you have underlying health conditions or are taking other medications. Herbal remedies should complement, not replace, conventional treatments. Collaboration with healthcare providers ensures these remedies are safely integrated into the overall management plan. Regular check-ins and adjustments to the plan are necessary to optimize yeast infection healing and overall well-being.

Medicinal Resources

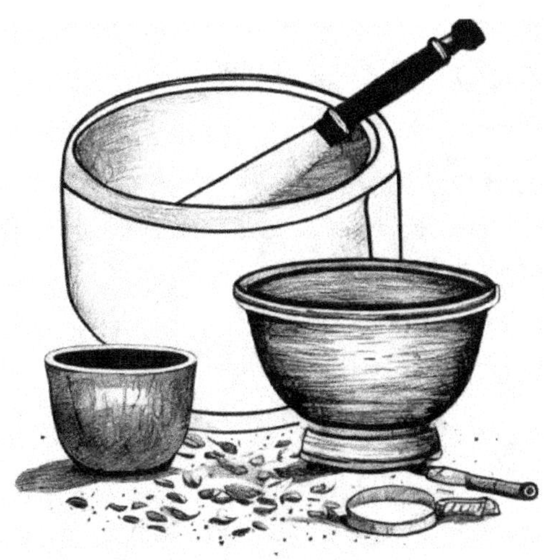

Herbs and Plants: These botanical species can be grown and harvested. These plants have various uses, including culinary, therapeutic, or ornamental.

Supplements: Some items are supplements or natural compounds that are often consumed for their potential health benefits. They are not plants but are derived from natural sources.

Natural Products: Items like "Honey," "Prunes and Prune Juice," and "Tea Tree Oil" are natural products. Honey is a natural sweetener bees produce, prunes are dried plums, and tea tree oil is an essential oil extracted from the tea tree leaves. While herbs and plants can be grown and harvested, supplements and natural products are typically not grown but can be purchased for various purposes.

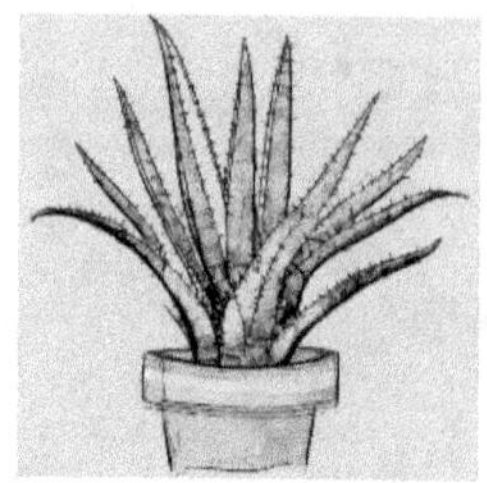

Aloe Vera (Aloe barbadensis miller) is a succulent plant with a long history of medicinal use. It is known for its gel, which is used for various health and skincare purposes. Here is a detailed overview of its historical use, medical uses, visual identification, growth conditions, care, propagation, harvesting, preservation, and preparation for medicinal use, along with precautions.

Historical Use: Aloe Vera has a rich history of medicinal use dating back thousands of years. It is believed to have originated in the Arabian Peninsula but has been cultivated and used worldwide. Ancient Egyptians called it the "plant of immortality" and used it for various health and skincare purposes. It has been used topically to treat skin conditions, wounds, and burns.

Medicinal Properties: Skin Conditions: Aloe Vera gel is commonly used to soothe and treat minor burns, sunburn, and skin irritations. Wound Healing: Aloe Vera accelerates wound healing and helps reduce scarring. Skin Moisturizer: Aloe Vera is a natural moisturizer for the skin. Oral Use: Some people use Aloe Vera internally for conditions like constipation, although this use is not recommended without medical supervision.

Visual Identification: Aloe Vera plants typically have the following characteristics: Thick, succulent, green leaves with serrated edges.
Leaves can grow up to 18-24 inches long and 2-4 inches wide. A gel-filled inner portion of the leaves. A rosette growth pattern. Tubular yellow or orange flowers on tall stalks.

Growth Conditions: US Zones: Aloe Vera can be grown outdoors in USDA hardiness zones 9-11. Time of Year: Aloe Vera is typically grown year-round in warm climates. Ideal Conditions and Soil Type for Growth: Light: Aloe Vera requires bright, indirect sunlight or partial shade. Temperature: It prefers temperatures between 59-77°F (15-25°C). Soil: Well-draining soil mix, such as a cactus or succulent potting mix. Water: Water sparingly, allowing the soil to dry out between watering. Container: It can be grown in containers or planted in well-draining soil in the ground.

Caring, Maintaining, and Pest Susceptibility: Water sparingly, as overwatering can lead to root rot. Fertilize sparingly, about once a month, during the growing season. Prune damaged or dead leaves. Aloe Vera is resistant to most pests but watch for mealybugs and scale insects.

Propagation Instructions: Aloe Vera can be propagated through offsets or "pups" that grow at the mother plant's base. Here is how: Carefully remove the offsets when they are a few inches tall.
Let them air dry for a day to form a callus Plant the balances in a small pot with well-drained soil. Water lightly and keep the new plants in indirect sunlight. Harvesting Instructions: You can harvest Aloe Vera leaves as needed for their gel. Select mature leaves from the outer part of the plant Use a sharp knife to cut the leaves close to the base. Store the harvested leaves in the refrigerator if you do not plan to use them immediately.

Preservation Techniques: Aloe Vera gel can be preserved in the following ways: Freezing: You can freeze Aloe Vera gel in ice cube trays for longer-term storage. Refrigeration: Freshly harvested gel can be stored in the refrigerator for a few weeks.

Commercial Aloe Vera Products: Commercially available Aloe Vera gels and creams are often preserved for extended shelf life.

Preparation for Medicinal Use: To use Aloe Vera for skin conditions, cut a leaf open and apply the gel directly to the affected area. It is essential to consult a healthcare professional or herbalist for internal use. Internal use can cause side effects and interactions with medications.

Possible Interactions or Precautions: Aloe Vera is safe for topical use but can cause skin irritation in some people. Internal use of Aloe Vera should be done under the guidance of a healthcare professional, as it may interact with medications and cause gastrointestinal discomfort.

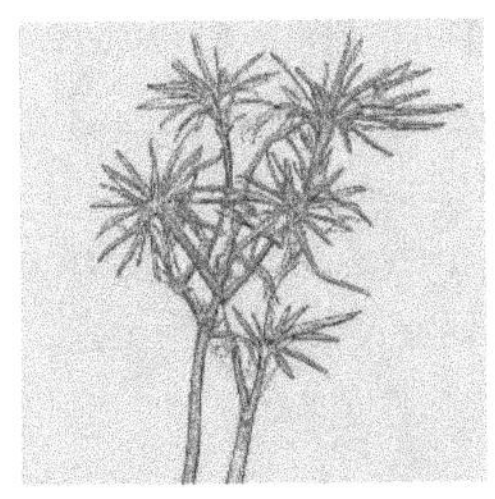

Anise (Pimpinella anisum) is an aromatic herb that has been used for various culinary and medicinal purposes for centuries. Here is a detailed overview of its historical use, current medically proven uses, visual identification, growth conditions, care, propagation, harvesting, preservation, preparation for medicinal use, and precautions.

Historical Use: Anise has a long history of use, dating back to ancient civilizations such as the Egyptians and Romans. It was traditionally used for its digestive and medicinal properties and as a spice in cooking. Anise seeds were also used as a breath freshener.

Medicinal Properties: Digestive Aid: Anise is commonly used to alleviate digestive discomfort, such as gas, bloating, and indigestion. Respiratory Health: Anise may help with coughs and respiratory conditions due to its expectorant properties. Menstrual Discomfort: It relieves menstrual cramps and regulates the menstrual cycle. Flavoring: Anise is used in various food and beverage products as a flavoring agent.

Visual Identification: Anise plants can be recognized by the following characteristics. Anise is an annual herb that can grow up to 2-3 feet in height. The leaves are feathery and finely divided.
Small white flowers grow in umbrella-like clusters. The seeds, which are the part used medicinally, are small, oval, and ridged.

Where it Grows, Zones, and Time of Year: Anise is typically grown in temperate climates and can be cultivated annually in many regions. It can be grown in USDA hardiness zones 4-9. Anise should be sown in the spring or early summer when the weather is warm. Ideal Conditions and Soil Type for Growth: Sunlight: Anise prefers full sun but can tolerate light shade. Temperature: It thrives in warm temperatures. Soil: Well-draining soil with a pH of 5.5-6.5 is ideal. Water: Anise plants need regular watering to moisten the earth but not waterlogged.

Caring, Maintaining, and Pest Susceptibility: Anise requires consistent moisture, and keeping the soil evenly moist is essential.

Use organic mulch to help maintain moisture and deter weeds. Anise may be susceptible to aphids, so monitor for infestations and address them promptly. Propagation Instructions: Anise can be propagated from seeds. Here is how: Sow anise seeds directly into the garden in early spring or early summer. Plant seeds about 1/4 inch deep, spaced 6-12 inches apart in rows. Keep the soil consistently moist. Seeds should germinate within a couple of   weeks.

Harvesting Instructions: Harvest anise seeds when they are fully mature, and the plant has gone to seed. Cut the seed heads and place them in a paper bag to dry. The seeds will naturally fall from the seed heads as they dry.

Preservation Techniques: To preserve anise seeds, follow these steps: Dry them thoroughly by spreading them out on a clean, dry surface away from direct sunlight. Once completely dry, store the seeds in an airtight container in a cool, dark place. Properly stored, anise seeds can remain flavorful for up to a year.

How to Prepare for Medicinal Use: For medicinal use, anise seeds are often used to make tea: Crush 1-2 teaspoons of anise seeds.
Place the crushed seeds in a cup and pour boiling water over them.
Cover and steep for 10-15 minutes. Strain the tea and drink it to relieve digestive discomfort or respiratory issues.

Possible Interactions and Precautions: Anise is considered safe when used in moderation. However, excessive use may lead to side effects such as nausea and diarrhea. If you have allergies or are pregnant or nursing, consult a healthcare provider before using anise medicinally. Anise may interact with certain medications, so it is essential to consult with a healthcare professional if you are taking prescription drugs.

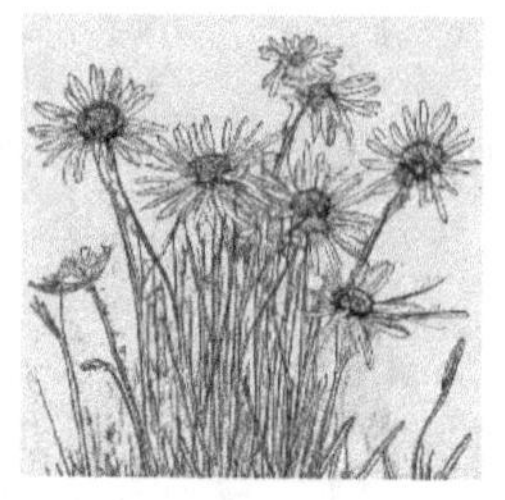

Arnica (Arnica montana) is a perennial herb with a long history of medicinal use. Here is a detailed overview of its historical use, current medically proven uses, visual identification, growth conditions, care, propagation, harvesting, preservation, preparation for medicinal use, and precautions.

Herbal preparations. Flowers are usually dried for later use.

Preservation Techniques: To preserve Arnica flowers, follow these steps: Dry them thoroughly by spreading them out on a clean, dry surface away from direct sunlight. Once completely dry, store the flowers in an airtight   container in a cool, dark place. Properly held, Arnica flowers can remain potent for several months.

Preparation for Medicinal Use: Arnica is primarily used topically. To make a soothing Arnica oil or ointment, Combine dried Arnica flowers with a carrier oil, such as olive oil. Allow the mixture to infuse for several weeks. Strain the oil and use it topically to relieve muscle aches, reduce inflammation, or soothe bruises.

Possible Interactions and Precautions: Arnica should only be used topically, as it can be toxic when ingested. Avoid internal use.
Do not apply Arnica to broken skin or open wounds. Allergic reactions to Arnica can occur, so a patch test is recommended before applying it to a larger skin area. Consult a healthcare provider before using Arnica, especially if you have sensitive skin or existing health conditions.

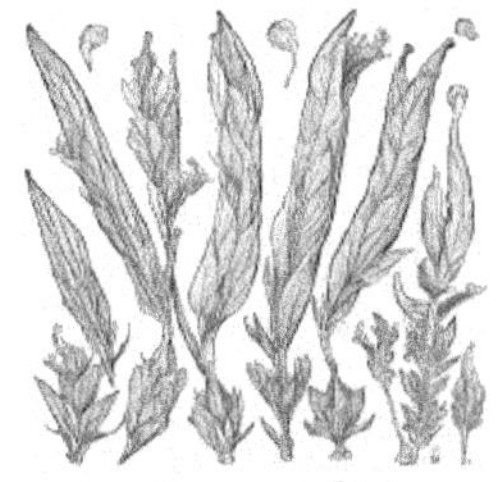 **Ashwagandha (Withania somnifera)** is an adaptogenic herb with a long history of use in traditional Ayurvedic medicine. Here is a detailed overview of its historical use, current medically proven uses, visual identification, growth conditions, care, propagation, harvesting, preservation, preparation for medicinal use, and precautions.

Historical Use: For centuries, Ashwagandha has been used in traditional Ayurvedic medicine for centuries to promote vitality, reduce stress, and support overall health and well-being. Its name translates to "smell of the horse" and is derived from the root's distinctive odor and the belief that consuming it can give you the strength and vitality of a horse.

Medicinal Properties: Ashwagandha is primarily used to combat stress, improve cognitive function, and boost energy. It is also known for its potential to manage anxiety and depression.

Visual Identification: Ashwagandha plants can be identified by the following characteristics: Small, greenish-yellow flowers. Simple leaves with an elliptic shape and a slightly hairy surface. Reddish-orange berries enclosed in papery pods. A central stem and a bushy growth habit.

Where it Grows, Zones, and Time of Year: Ashwagandha is native to the dry regions of India, the Middle East, and parts of Africa. It thrives in warm climates and can be grown in USDA hardiness zones 8-12. Ashwagandha is usually grown year-round in areas with warm temperatures.

Ideal Conditions and Soil Type for Growth: Light: Ashwagandha prefers full sun but can tolerate light shade. Temperature: It thrives in warm to hot conditions. Soil: Well-draining, sandy loam is ideal. Water: Keep the soil consistently moist, but do not overwater.

Caring, Maintaining, and Pest Susceptibility: Ashwagandha requires regular watering, especially in hot weather. Fertilize the plant with a balanced, all-purpose fertilizer during the growing season. Watch for common pests like aphids and spider mites.

Propagation Instructions: Ashwagandha can be propagated from seeds or cuttings. Here is how: For seeds, sow them in a well-prepared garden bed with sandy loam soil. Keep the soil consistently moist but not waterlogged. Seeds should germinate within a couple of weeks.

Harvesting Instructions: Ashwagandha roots are harvested for medicinal use. They are typically harvested after six months to a year of growth when the plant matures. Carefully dig up the roots, remove the soil, and clean them thoroughly.

Preservation Techniques: To preserve Ashwagandha roots, Clean the roots thoroughly to remove soil and debris. Allow the roots to air dry for a few days. Store the dried roots in an airtight container in a cool, dark place. Safely stored, Ashwagandha roots can remain potent for a year or more.

Preparation for Medicinal Use: Ashwagandha roots can be used to make various preparations, including powders, capsules, tinctures, and teas. The root is commonly dried and ground into a fine powder for ease of use. Consult with a healthcare provider or herbalist for appropriate form and dosage guidance.

Possible Interactions and Precautions: Ashwagandha is well-tolerated but may interact with certain medications, so consult a healthcare provider before use. Avoid Ashwagandha if you are pregnant or breastfeeding unless directed by a healthcare provider. Some people may experience mild side effects such as digestive upset, so start with a lower dose if you are trying it for the first time.

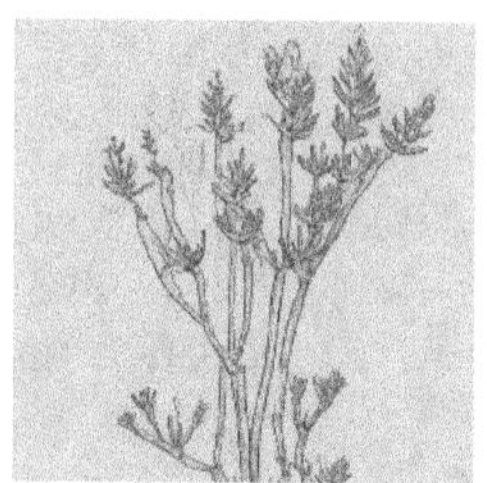

Astragalus (Astragalus membranaceus), also known as Huang Qi, is a popular medicinal herb in traditional Chinese medicine and has gained recognition in Western herbal medicine. Here is a detailed overview of its historical use, current medically proven services, visual identification, growth conditions, care, propagation, harvesting, preservation, preparation for medicinal use, and precautions.

Historical Use: Astragalus has a long history of use in traditional Chinese medicine, where it is considered a vital herb for supporting overall health and vitality. It was traditionally used to strengthen the body, boost the immune system, and improve longevity.

Medicinal Properties: Immune System Support: Astragalus is known for its immune-boosting properties. It can enhance the body's defense mechanisms and help prevent illness. Adaptogen: Astragalus acts as an adaptogen, helping the body cope with stress and maintain balance. Anti-Inflammatory: It has anti-inflammatory properties and may be used to reduce inflammation. Cardiovascular Health: Some studies suggest that astragalus may help support heart health and reduce high blood pressure.

Visual Identification: Astragalus plants can be recognized by the following characteristics: Small, shrub-like plants with multiple stems. Pinnate leaves with many leaflets. Clusters of small, pea-like flowers that are typically yellow. The root, which is the part used medicinally, is long and tapered with a yellowish-brown color.

Where it Grows, Zones, and Time of Year: Astragalus is native to northern China and Mongolia but is also cultivated in other regions. In the United States, it is grown in USDA hardiness zones 6-8 in the United States. Plant Astragalus in the spring or early summer when the soil is warm.

Ideal Conditions and Soil Type for Growth: Sunlight: Astragalus prefers full sun, but it can tolerate partial shade. Temperature: It thrives in warm climates and is drought tolerant. Soil: Well-draining, sandy, or loamy soil with a pH of 6.0-7.0 is ideal. Water: Provide consistent moisture but avoid overwatering.

Caring, Maintaining, and Pest Susceptibility: Water young plants regularly until established, then water as needed. Mulching around the base of the plant can help conserve moisture and reduce weed competition. Astragalus is resistant to pests and diseases.

Propagation Instructions: Astragalus can be propagated from seeds or by root division. To propagate from seeds: Collect ripe seeds in the fall. Scarify the seeds by lightly scratching their surface or soaking them in hot water. Plant the scarified seeds about 1/4 inch deep in well-draining soil. Keep the soil consistently moist, and the seeds should germinate in a few weeks.

Harvesting Instructions: Astragalus root is typically harvested in the fall or after the plant has reached 3-4 years of age. Dig up the roots carefully to avoid damaging them.

Preservation Techniques: To preserve astragalus roots, Clean the roots by removing dirt and debris. Dry the roots by spreading them out in a single layer in a well-ventilated area, away from direct sunlight. Once completely dry, store the roots in an airtight container in a cool, dark place. Properly stored, the astragalus root can last for several years.

How to Prepare for Medicinal Use: Astragalus root can be prepared as a decoction (strong tea) for medicinal use. Here is how: Cut the dried root into small pieces. Place 1-2 tablespoons of the root in a pot with 2-3 cups of water. Simmer the mixture for about 30 minutes to 1 hour. Strain and drink the decoction. The recommended dosage can vary, so consult with a healthcare professional.

Possible Interactions and Precautions: Astragalus is safe when used as directed. However, it may interact with certain medications or medical conditions, so consult a healthcare provider before using it, especially if you are pregnant, nursing, or have underlying health concerns. Astragalus should not be used as a replacement for professional medical treatment when dealing with serious health conditions.

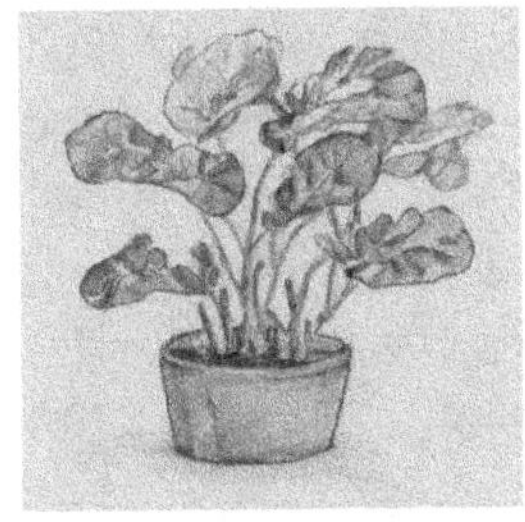 **Bacopa (Bacopa monnieri)**, also known as Brahmi, is a medicinal herb with a rich history of use in Ayurvedic medicine. Here is a detailed overview of its historical use, current medically proven uses, visual identification, growth conditions, care, propagation, harvesting, preservation, preparation for medicinal use, and precautions.

Historical Use: Bacopa has been used for centuries in Ayurvedic medicine, particularly for enhancing cognitive function, reducing anxiety, and promoting overall well-being. It is considered a powerful adaptogen and nootropic. Medicinal Properties: Cognitive Enhancement: Bacopa can potentially enhance memory, concentration, and cognitive function. It may help reduce stress and anxiety due to its adaptogenic properties. Neuroprotective: Bacopa may have neuroprotective effects, potentially slowing down the aging of brain cells. Anti-Inflammatory: It has anti-inflammatory properties that may benefit various health conditions. Visual Identification: Bacopa plants can be recognized by the following characteristics: Low-growing, creeping herb with small, succulent leaves. Leaves are oval-shaped, thick, and succulent, usually about 1 cm long. Small white or purple flowers with five petals. Grows as a ground cover in moist, wet, and marshy areas.

Where it Grows, Zones, and Time of Year: Bacopa is native to wetlands and marshy areas in tropical and subtropical regions. It is typically grown as an annual or indoor plant in zones 9-11 in the United States. Plant Bacopa in the spring or early summer when the weather is warm. Ideal Conditions and Soil Type for Growth: Sunlight: Bacopa prefers partial shade or filtered sunlight, especially in hot climates. Temperature: It thrives in warm to hot temperatures. Soil: Well-draining, nutrient-rich, and slightly acidic soil with a pH of 6.0-7.5. Water: Keep the soil consistently moist. Bacopa thrives in aquatic or semi-aquatic conditions. Caring, Maintaining, and Pest Susceptibility: Regularly water to moisten the soil but avoid waterlogging. Mulch around the base of the plant to conserve moisture and prevent weed competition. Bacopa is resistant to pests and diseases.

Propagation Instructions: Bacopa can be propagated through stem cuttings. Here is how: Take 4–6-inch cuttings from the tips of healthy Bacopa stems. Remove lower leaves from the cuttings.
Place the cuttings in a glass of water or a pot with well-draining soil. Keep the soil or water consistently moist. Once roots develop, transplant the cuttings into a larger container or garden.

Harvesting Instructions: For medicinal use, harvest Bacopa leaves when they are mature, usually after 3-4 months of growth. Simply trim the leaves from the stems as needed.

Preservation Techniques: To preserve Bacopa leaves, Wash the leaves thoroughly to remove any dirt or debris. Dry the leaves by spreading them out on a clean, dry surface away from direct sunlight. Once completely dry, store the leaves in an airtight container in a cool, dark place. Properly stored, Bacopa leaves can retain their potency for several months.

How to Prepare for Medicinal Use: Bacopa leaves are commonly consumed as tea or in capsules for medicinal use. To make Bacopa tea, use 1-2 teaspoons of dried Bacopa leaves. Boil water and pour it over the leaves in a cup. Cover and steep for 5-10 minutes. Strain the tea and drink. The recommended dosage can vary, so consult with a healthcare professional. Possible

Interactions and Precautions: Bacopa is considered safe when used as directed, but it may interact with certain medications, especially those for diabetes, blood pressure, and sedatives. Pregnant and nursing women and individuals with certain medical conditions should consult a healthcare provider before using Bacopa. Discontinue use if you experience adverse effects and consult with a healthcare professional.

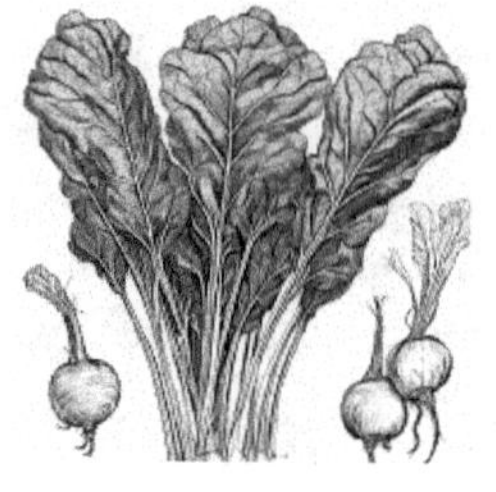

Beetroot (Beta vulgaris) is a versatile and nutritious vegetable that has been consumed for its health benefits and culinary uses for centuries. Here is a detailed overview of beetroot, including its historical use, nutritional value, preparation, cooking methods, and potential health benefits.

Historical Use: Beetroot has a long consumption history, dating back to ancient civilizations, including the Greeks and Romans. Originally, beetroot was cultivated for its leaves, which are edible and nutritious. Over time, its vibrant, earthy-tasting root gained popularity as a food source and later as a natural food coloring.

Nutritional Value: Beetroot is rich in essential nutrients and antioxidants, making it a healthy addition to your diet. Here are some key components of its nutritional value: Vitamins and Minerals: Beetroot is a useful source of essential vitamins and minerals, including vitamin C, folate (vitamin B9), potassium, and manganese. Dietary Fiber: Beetroot contains dietary fiber, which supports digestion and can help maintain a healthy gut. Antioxidants Beetroots are rich in antioxidants, such as betalains, which have anti-inflammatory and potential anti-cancer properties.

Preparation: When preparing beetroot, washing, and peeling it to remove any residual dirt is essential. Beetroot leaves, stems, and roots are all edible, so that you can incorporate various parts of the plant into your meals. Some common ways to prepare beetroot include Raw: Grated beetroot can be used in salads for added crunch and color. Roasted: Roasted beetroot makes a sweet and tender side dish. Boiled: Boiled beetroot is versatile and can be used in various dishes, such as soups and stews. Pickled: Pickled beetroot adds a tangy and flavorful element to salads and sandwiches.

Cooking Methods: Beetroot can be cooked in several ways, depending on your preference. Roasting: Roasting beetroot enhances its natural sweetness and flavor. Cover the beetroot in olive oil, salt, and pepper, wrap it in foil, and roast in the oven until tender.

Boiling: Boiled beetroot is tender and can be sliced or diced for use in various recipes. To boil beetroot, scrub them, place them in a pot of water, and cook until they are easily pierced with a fork.
Steaming: Steamed beetroot retains more of its nutrients compared to boiling. Steam whole or sliced beetroot until tender.
Grilling: Grilled beetroot has a smoky flavor and is a unique addition to a barbecue.

Health Benefits: Beetroot offers several potential health benefits, including Blood Pressure. The nitrates in beetroot may help lower blood pressure when consumed regularly. Digestive Health: Beetroot's fiber content supports healthy digestion. Antioxidant Properties: The antioxidants in beetroot can help reduce inflammation and oxidative stress. Athletic Performance: Some studies suggest that beetroot juice can improve endurance and exercise performance due to its nitrate content. Detoxification: Beetroot supports liver health and may aid in detoxification processes. It is essential to include beetroot as part of a balanced diet to enjoy these potential health benefits fully.

Precautions: Beetroot can cause red or pink urine and stools due to its natural pigments, which are harmless. People with kidney problems may want to consume beetroot in moderation due to its high oxalate.

Berberine (Berberis vulgaris) Berberine is a naturally occurring compound found in several plants. Such as Goldenseal (Hydrastis canadensis) and Oregon grape (Mahonia aquifolium). It has a long history of use in traditional medicine, particularly in Chinese and Ayurvedic traditions, and has gained recognition for its potential medical benefits in contemporary research. Here is a detailed overview of its uses, sources, preparation, and precautions:

Historical Use: Berberine has been used for centuries in traditional medicine systems. In Chinese medicine, it is used for its antimicrobial, anti-inflammatory, and digestive properties. It has been used to treat various conditions, including diarrhea, fungal infections, and gastrointestinal disorders.

Medicinal Properties: Blood Sugar Control: Berberine has been studied for its potential to help regulate blood sugar levels and improve insulin sensitivity, making it a potential treatment for type 2 diabetes. Cholesterol Management: It may help lower LDL ("bad") cholesterol levels, which benefits heart health. Antimicrobial Properties: Berberine exhibits antimicrobial effects against bacteria, fungi, and parasites. Anti-Inflammatory: It has anti-inflammatory properties and may be used to manage certain inflammatory conditions.

Sources: Berberine is primarily sourced from the following plants:
Goldenseal (Hydrastis canadensis): Native to North America, goldenseal has been a traditional source of berberine. Barberry (Berberis vulgaris): The bark and roots of this plant are rich in

berberine. Oregon Grape (Mahonia aquifolium): The roots and bark of this plant are another source of berberine.

Preparation: Berberine can be obtained as a supplement in capsules or tablets. The dosage can vary, so following the recommended guidelines on the product label or consulting with a healthcare professional for personalized recommendations is essential.

Possible Interactions and Precautions: Berberine may interact with certain medications, including blood-thinning medications, medications for high blood pressure, and others. Consult a healthcare provider before using Berberine if you are taking prescription medications. Pregnant or nursing women and individuals with certain medical conditions, such as liver or kidney disease, should consult a healthcare professional before using Berberine. In some individuals, Berberine may cause gastrointestinal side effects such as diarrhea, cramping, and flatulence. It is advisable to start with a lower dose and gradually increase it to assess tolerance. Use berberine supplements from reputable sources to ensure product quality and safety.

Please note that while berberine has shown promise in various areas of health, research is ongoing, and it should not be used as a replacement for professional medical treatment. Always consult a healthcare provider before starting any new supplement or treatment regimen.

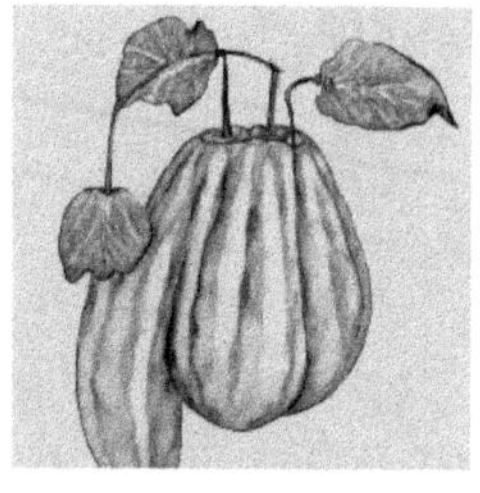

Bitter Melon (Momordica charantia) is a unique fruit with a long history of use in traditional medicine and culinary traditions. Here is a detailed overview of its historical use, current medically proven benefits, visual identification, growth conditions, care, preparation for culinary use, and precautions.

Historical Use: Bitter Melon has been used for centuries in traditional medicine, particularly in Asia, Africa, and the Caribbean. It has been employed to treat various conditions, including diabetes gastrointestinal issues, and as a general health tonic.

Medicinal Properties: Diabetes Management: Bitter Melon is known for its potential to lower blood sugar levels. It contains compounds that mimic the action of insulin, making it helpful in managing diabetes. Antioxidant Properties: Bitter Melon includes antioxidants that help combat oxidative stress and reduce inflammation. Weight Management: It may aid in weight management by supporting metabolism and fat reduction. Immune Support: Some studies suggest that Bitter Melon may help enhance the immune system.

Visual Identification: Bitter Melon plants can be recognized by the following characteristics: Vine-like plants with deeply lobed leaves and elongated, warty fruit that can vary in size and color (green, yellow, or orange). Flowers are typically yellow and have both male and female flowers on the same plant.

Growth Conditions: Bitter Melon can be grown in warm, tropical, and subtropical climates. It thrives in regions with consistently elevated temperatures and ample sunlight.

Care: Provide a trellis or support structure for the vine to climb. Bitter Melon plants require well-drained, fertile soil. Adequate watering is essential, especially during dry periods. Regular pruning may be necessary to manage the growth and encourage fruit production.

Preparation for Culinary Use: Bitter Melon is often used in various culinary dishes. Here is how to prepare it: Slice the Bitter Melon lengthwise and remove the seeds and pith. Slice the fruit into thin rounds or strips. To reduce its bitterness, soak the slices in salted water for 15-30 minutes and then rinse. Bitter Melon can be used in stir-fries, curries, soups, or salads. Cooking with other ingredients can help balance its bitter taste.

Precautions: Bitter Melon is not recommended for individuals with hypoglycemia or those taking medications for low blood sugar. Pregnant or nursing women should avoid excessive consumption of Bitter Melon, as it may have adverse effects. Bitter Melon's bitter taste can be unpalatable to some, so it is important to use it in moderation and consider its preparation to reduce bitterness.

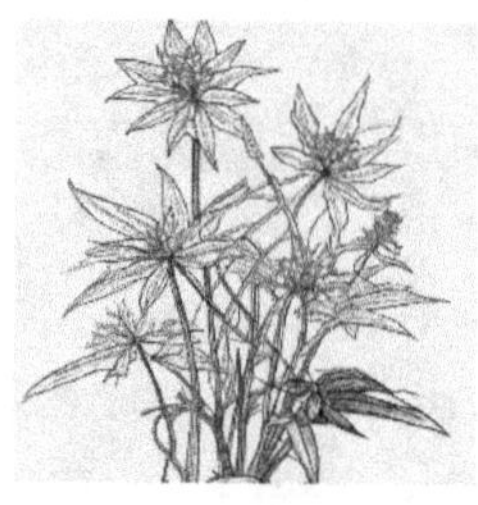

Black Cohosh (Actaea racemosa), also known as Cimicifuga racemosa, is an herbaceous plant native to eastern North America. It has a long history of use in traditional medicine and has been the subject of scientific research to understand its potential medical uses. Here is a detailed overview of its historical use, current medically proven uses, visual identification, growth conditions, care, preparation for medicinal use, and precautions.

Historical Use: Black Cohosh has a history of medicinal use by Indigenous peoples in North America, including relief from menstrual discomfort and childbirth pain. It was later adopted in traditional medicine systems and has been used for a variety of ailments, including menopausal symptoms.

Medicinal Properties: Menopausal Symptom Relief: Black Cohosh is commonly used to alleviate menopausal symptoms such as hot flashes, night sweats, mood swings, and sleep disturbances.
Menstrual Symptom Relief: It may help alleviate menstrual discomfort, including cramps. Anti-Inflammatory: Black Cohosh has shown anti-inflammatory properties, which may be useful for inflammation-related conditions.

Visual Identification: Black Cohosh plants can be recognized by the following characteristics: tall, slender stems with a feathery cluster of white flowers at the top. Leaves are compounded with several deeply lobed leaflets. The plant produces a spike of white, bottlebrush-like flowers. Black Cohosh grows 3 to 8 feet in height.

Growth Conditions: Black Cohosh is native to eastern North America and can be found in hardwood forests and along stream banks. It typically grows in USDA hardiness zones 3-8.

Care: Black Cohosh prefers partial to full shade and well-draining, humus-rich soil. Keep the soil consistently moist but not waterlogged. Regularly mulch around the plant to maintain soil moisture and reduce weed competition.

Preparation for Medicinal Use: Black Cohosh is commonly used as a tincture or capsule. The dried rhizome and root of the plant are used to prepare these products. Here is how to make a tincture: Clean and chop the dried rhizome and root into small pieces. Place the chopped plant material in a glass jar. Cover the plant material with a high-proof alcohol (such as vodka or brandy). Seal the jar and store it in a cool, dark place for about 4-6 weeks, shaking it daily. Strain the liquid through a fine mesh or cheesecloth and transfer it to a dark glass tincture bottle. The recommended dosage can vary, so consult a healthcare professional for guidance.

Precautions: Consult with a healthcare provider before using Black Cohosh, especially if you are pregnant, nursing, or have any underlying health concerns. Some individuals may experience side effects, including gastrointestinal discomfort or headaches, while using Black Cohosh. If adverse reactions occur, discontinue use. Use Black Cohosh for a specific duration and follow recommended dosages. Prolonged use may lead to liver toxicity, so monitoring is essential. Black Cohosh may interact with certain medications, so consult a healthcare provider if you take prescription drugs.

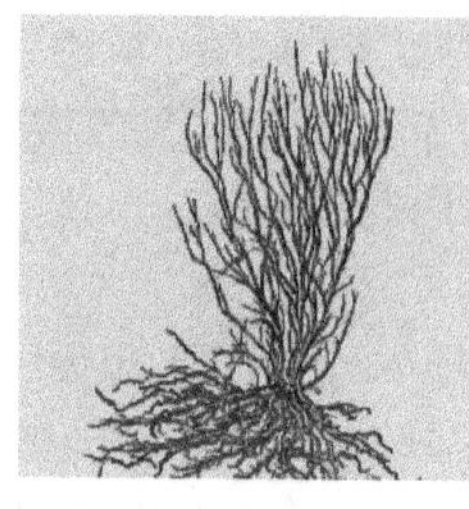

Bladderwrack (Fucus vesiculosus) is a brown seaweed growing in coastal regions, particularly in the Northern Hemisphere. It has been used for centuries in traditional medicine, particularly in coastal communities, and is a rich source of various nutrients. Here is a detailed overview of its historical use, current medically proven uses, visual identification, growth conditions, care, preparation for medicinal use, and precautions.

Historical Use: Bladderwrack has a long history of use, primarily in traditional coastal communities and herbal medicine systems. It was used to treat various health conditions and is known for its nutrient-rich content.

Medicinal Properties: Iodine Source: Bladderwrack is a natural iodine source essential for proper thyroid function. Nutrient-rich: It is rich in vitamins, minerals, and antioxidants, which can support overall health. Anti-Inflammatory: Bladderwrack contains compounds that have anti-inflammatory properties.

Visual Identification: Bladderwrack can be recognized by the following characteristics: Olive-green to deep brown, frond-like structure with air bladders. The air bladders give the seaweed its name, as they resemble small bladders or sacs. It attaches to rocks or other substrates with a holdfast and can be found in intertidal zones.

Growth Conditions: Bladderwrack grows in cold, temperate waters along rocky coastlines. It can be found in the Northern Hemisphere, particularly in the North Atlantic and North Pacific oceans.

Care: Bladderwrack is a marine plant and typically grows in natural habitats. It is not commonly cultivated in gardens. Protecting and conserving these habitats is important if you have access to a coastal area where it naturally grows.

Preparation for Medicinal Use: Bladderwrack can be prepared for medicinal use in several ways: Dried Seaweed: You can dry the seaweed and grind it into a powder to be used in capsules or added to smoothies or food. Tincture: Some herbalists prepare Bladderwrack tinctures using alcohol or glycerin. Topical Use: Bladderwrack can be used topically in creams, gels, or poultices for skin-related issues.

Precautions: If you are considering using Bladderwrack for its iodine content, consult a healthcare provider to ensure you get the appropriate dose, as excessive iodine intake can have adverse effects. Be cautious about foraging for Bladderwrack in the wild, as it is important to know the specific coastal regulations and guidelines for sustainable harvesting and to ensure that the waters where it is collected are free from contamination. It is essential to source Bladderwrack from reputable suppliers to ensure it is free from pollutants and heavy metals. If you have underlying health conditions, are pregnant, nursing, or taking medications, consult with a healthcare provider before using Bladderwrack medicinally.

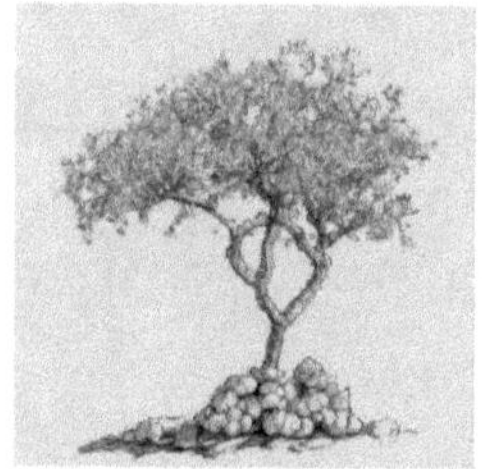

Boswellia (Boswellia serrata), also known as Indian frankincense, is a resin obtained from the Boswellia serrata tree. It has a long history of use in traditional medicine and has been researched for its potential health benefits. Here is a detailed overview of its historical use, current medically proven uses, visual identification, growth conditions, care, preparation for medicinal use, and precautions. Historical Use: Boswellia has been used in traditional Ayurvedic and traditional Chinese medicine for thousands of years. It was traditionally used for its anti-inflammatory and analgesic properties and as a remedy for various health conditions.

Medicinal Properties: Anti-Inflammatory Properties: Boswellia contains compounds such as Boswellia acids that have anti-inflammatory effects. It reduces inflammation and manages conditions like osteoarthritis and inflammatory bowel disease. Joint Health: It is often used to alleviate pain and improve mobility. Asthma: Some studies suggest that Boswellia may positively impact bronchial asthma. Inflammatory Bowel Disease: It is sometimes used to help manage the symptoms of conditions like ulcerative colitis and Crohn's disease.

Visual Identification: Boswellia serrata is a small to medium-sized deciduous tree that can reach about twenty feet. It has distinctive palmate leaves and a smooth, papery bark. The tree produces small, greenish-white flowers and woody capsules containing resin.

Growth Conditions: Boswellia serrata is native to India, the Middle East, and North Africa. It thrives in arid and semi-arid regions and prefers well-drained, rocky soil. It is well-adapted to dry, tropical climates.

Care: Boswellia trees are typically grown in their natural habitat and require minimal maintenance. In their native regions, they can be found growing in the wild.

Preparation for Medicinal Use: Boswellia resin is a part of the plant used for medicinal purposes. It is available in various forms, including capsules, powders, and extracts. The recommended dosage can vary based on the specific health condition being addressed. Following the instructions on the product label or consulting with a healthcare provider for personalized Recommendations is essential.

Precautions:
Boswellia is considered safe when used as directed. However, it may interact with certain medications, including blood-thinning drugs. Consult a healthcare provider before using Boswellia, especially if taking prescriptions.

Medications.
Pregnant or nursing women and individuals with certain medical conditions should consult a healthcare professional before using Boswellia. While Boswellia is well-tolerated by most people, some may experience minor gastrointestinal discomfort or skin rashes. If adverse reactions occur, discontinue use, and consult with a healthcare provider.

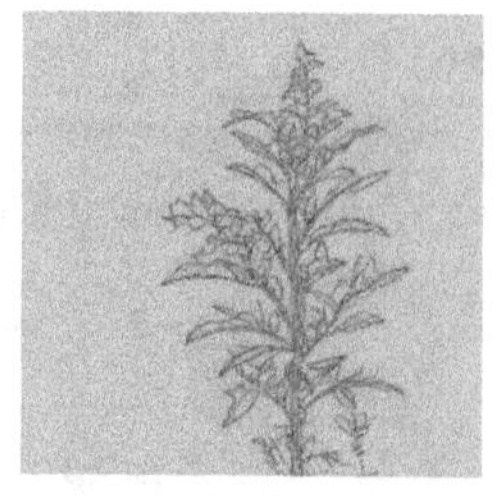

Buchu (Agathosma betulina),

also known as round leaf buchu, is a plant native to South Africa. It has been used for centuries by Indigenous peoples and in traditional herbal medicine for various medicinal purposes. Here is a detailed overview of its historical use, current medically proven uses, visual identification, growth conditions, care, preparation for medicinal use, and precautions: Historical Use: Buchu has a long history of use by indigenous groups in South Africa, where it was traditionally used for its diuretic, anti-inflammatory, and antispasmodic properties. It also treated urinary tract infections, stomach complaints, and rheumatism.

Medicinal Properties: Urinary Health: Buchu alleviates urinary tract infections and promotes overall urinary health. Anti-Inflammatory: It has anti-inflammatory properties and may be used for inflammation-related conditions. Antispasmodic: Buchu may help relieve muscle spasms and cramps. Diuretic: It is known for its diuretic effect, helping to increase urine production and remove excess fluids from the body.

Visual Identification: Buchu plants can be recognized by the following characteristics: Small, aromatic shrubs with round, glossy leaves. When crushed, the leaves are dotted with oil glands that release a distinctive fragrance. The plant produces small white to pink flowers. Buchu leaves are typically harvested for medicinal use.

Growth Conditions: Buchu is native to the Western Cape region of South Africa. It thrives in the fynbos biome, characterized by a Mediterranean climate with wet winters and dry summers.

Care: Buchu is typically grown in its native habitat in South Africa and is not commonly cultivated in gardens. It requires specific environmental conditions to thrive.

Preparation for Medicinal Use: Buchu is available in various forms, including dried leaves, capsules, teas, and tinctures. The dried leaves can be used to prepare herbal tea. Here is how to make Buchu tea: Use about 1-2 teaspoons of dried Buchu leaves. Boil water and pour it over the leaves in a cup. Cover and steep for 5-10 minutes. Strain the tea and drink. The recommended dosage can vary, so consult a healthcare professional for guidance.

Precautions:
Buchu is considered safe when used as directed. However, it may interact with certain medications, especially diuretics and lithium. Consult with a healthcare provider before using Buchu, especially if taking prescription medications. Pregnant or nursing women and individuals with certain medical conditions should consult with a healthcare professional before using Buchu. Buchu should not be used as a replacement for professional medical treatment when dealing with serious health conditions.

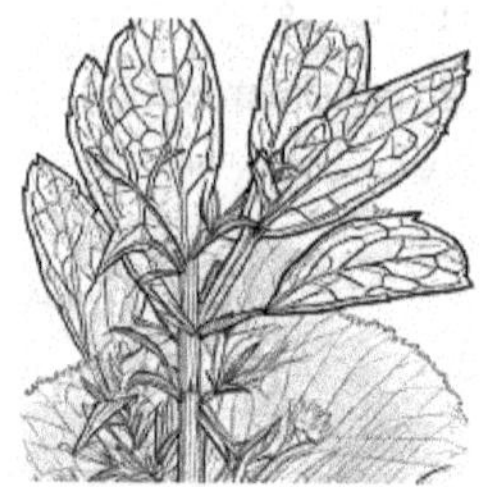

Bugleweed (Lycopus virginicus) is an herbaceous perennial plant that has been used for its potential medicinal properties for various health concerns. Here is a detailed overview of bugleweed, including its historical use, medicinal uses, visual identification, growth conditions, preparation, and potential health benefits.

Historical Use: Bugleweed has a history of traditional use among Indigenous peoples and early European settlers. It was used for various medicinal purposes, particularly to address conditions related to the respiratory and cardiovascular systems.

Medicinal Uses: Bugleweed is believed to have potential health benefits and has been used for various purposes, including Respiratory Conditions. Bugleweed is traditionally used to relieve symptoms of respiratory ailments, such as coughs and Bronchitis. Cardiovascular Health: Some believe that bugleweed may help support cardiovascular health and manage mild heart Palpitations. Thyroid Health: Bugleweed has been studied for its potential role in managing hyperthyroidism, a condition characterized by an overactive thyroid gland.

Visual Identification: Bugleweed plants typically have the following characteristics: Bugleweed is a low-growing plant, usually reaching a height of about 6-12 inches (15-30 cm). It features square stems with leaves that are opposite, lance-shaped, and serrated. The leaves of bugleweed can vary in color, ranging from dark green to reddish-purple, depending on the variety. It produces spikes of small, tubular flowers that can be white, pink, or purple.

Growth Conditions: Bugleweed grows well under specific conditions. Some key factors to consider when cultivating bugleweed: US Zones: Bugleweed can be grown in USDA hardiness zones 3-8, depending on the variety.

Ideal Soil: Bugleweed prefers well-draining soil and can tolerate a range of soil types, including sandy, loamy, or clay soils. Soil pH should be slightly acidic to neutral. Light: Bugleweed thrives in partial to full shade, making it an excellent choice for shaded or woodland gardens. Water: Keep the soil consistently moist, particularly during hot and dry conditions.

Preparation and Health Benefits: The aerial parts of bugleweed (leaves and flowers) make teas, tinctures, or extracts. Here is how you can prepare and benefit from bugleweed: Tea: Infusing dried or fresh bugleweed leaves in hot water can create a tea that some people use to alleviate respiratory discomfort or calm mild heart   palpitations.

Tinctures and Extracts: Liquid preparations of bugleweed can be taken as directed to support specific health concerns. It is essential to consult with a healthcare provider before using bugleweed for medicinal purposes, especially if you have pre-existing health conditions or are taking other medications. While bugleweed shows promise in addressing certain health issues, its effectiveness can vary among individuals.

Precautions: Bugleweed is safe when used as recommended. However, there are a few precautions to consider: Allergic Reactions: Some individuals may experience allergic reactions to bugleweed. If you are sensitive to members of the mint family (Lamiaceae), which bugleweed belongs to, use it with caution.

Thyroid Disorders: Bugleweed's potential to affect thyroid function should be carefully monitored by healthcare professionals, especially if you have thyroid disorders.

Dosage: Ensure you follow recommended dosages when using bugleweed supplements or preparations. Overuse can lead to side effects.

Interactions:
Consult a healthcare provider, especially if you are taking medications or have underlying health issues, as bugleweed may interact with certain drugs or health conditions. As with any herbal remedy, it is advisable to consult with a healthcare provider, herbalist, or qualified practitioner to determine the appropriateness of bugleweed for your specific health needs.

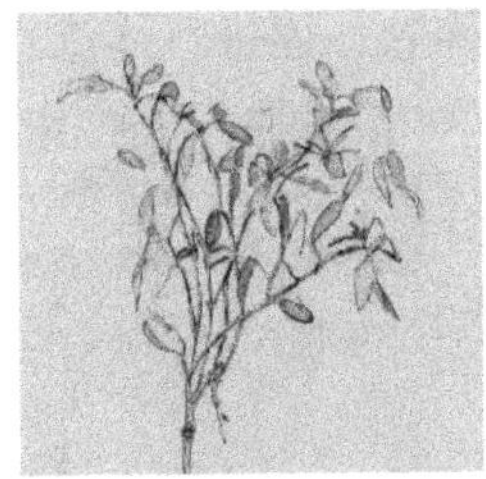

Butcher's Broom (Ruscus aculeatus) is a small evergreen shrub native to Mediterranean regions and some parts of Europe. It has a long history of use in traditional herbal medicine and has been researched for its potential medicinal properties. Here is a detailed overview of its historical use, current medically proven uses, visual identification, growth conditions, care, preparation for medicinal use, and precautions.

Historical Use: Butcher's Broom has been used for centuries in traditional European herbal medicine. It was traditionally used for its diuretic, laxative, and anti-inflammatory properties and as a remedy for various health conditions, including hemorrhoids and varicose veins.

Medicinal Properties: Vascular Health: Butcher's Broom is commonly used to support vascular health and improve circulation. It may help alleviate chronic venous insufficiency (CVI) symptoms, such as leg swelling and discomfort. Anti-Inflammatory: It has anti-inflammatory properties and may be used to manage inflammation-related conditions. Hemorrhoids: Butcher's Broom may be used to relieve symptoms of hemorrhoids, including pain and swelling.

Lymphedema: Some studies suggest that Butcher's Broom may be beneficial for managing lymphedema.

Visual Identification: Butcher's Broom can be recognized by the following characteristics: Low-growing evergreen shrub with tough, spine-tipped leaves that resemble flattened stems. Small, inconspicuous greenish-white flowers are produced in the center of the leaf cluster. Red berries are produced, which are not typically used medicinally.

Growth Conditions: Butcher's Broom is native to Mediterranean regions and prefers well-drained, sandy, or loamy soil. It is typically found in woodland and scrubland habitats.

Care: Butcher's Broom is low-maintenance and can be grown in gardens. It prefers partial to full shade and well-draining soil. It is drought-tolerant once established.

Preparation for Medicinal Use: Butcher's Broom is available in various forms, including capsules, tinctures, and ointments. The root of the plant is typically used for its medicinal properties. The recommended dosage can vary, so follow the product label instructions or consult a healthcare professional for personalized recommendations.

Precautions: Butcher's Broom is considered safe when used as directed. However, it may interact with certain medications, including blood-thinning drugs. Consult with a healthcare provider before using Butcher's Broom, especially if taking prescription medications.

Pregnant or nursing women and individuals with certain medical conditions should consult a healthcare professional before using Butcher's Broom. While Butcher's Broom has potential health benefits, it should not replace professional medical treatment when dealing with serious health conditions.

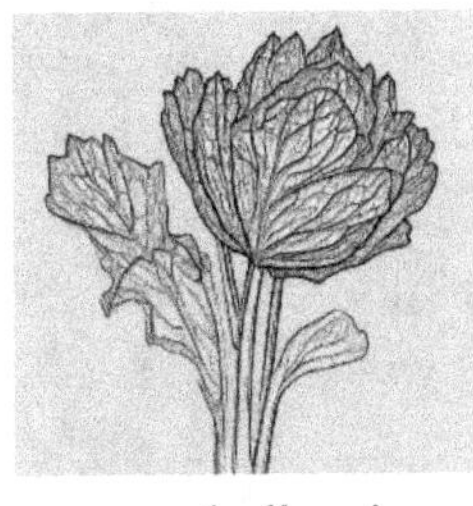

Butterbur (Petasites hybridus)

is a perennial plant used in traditional herbal medicine for centuries, primarily in Europe and Asia. It has been researched for its potential medicinal properties, particularly for managing migraines and seasonal allergies.

Historical Use: Butterbur has a long history of use in traditional European and Asian herbal medicine. It was traditionally used to treat various health conditions, including fever, asthma, and digestive issues.

Medicinal Properties: Migraine Prevention: Butterbur has shown promise in reducing the frequency and severity of migraines in some individuals. Allergy Relief: It may be used to alleviate symptoms of seasonal allergies, such as hay fever. It is believed to work by reducing the release of histamines. Anti-Inflammatory: Butterbur has anti-inflammatory properties and may be used to manage conditions associated with inflammation.

Visual Identification: Butterbur plants can be recognized by the following characteristics: Large, heart-shaped leaves with a serrated edge. Pink, purplish, or white flower clusters that appear before the leaves. The plant typically grows in damp or marshy areas.

Growth Conditions: Butterbur prefers moist, marshy, and shady habitats, often found in wetlands or along riverbanks. It is native to Europe and parts of Asia.

Care:
Butterbur is not commonly cultivated in gardens, as it prefers specific environmental conditions that are difficult to replicate. If you plan to grow Butterbur, it is essential to mimic its natural habitat, providing damp, shady areas with rich, well-drained soil.

Preparation for Medicinal Use: Butterbur is available in various forms, including capsules, tablets, and extracts. The root and rhizome are typically used for their medicinal properties. The recommended dosage can vary, so following the instructions on the product label or consulting with a healthcare professional for personalized recommendations is important.

Precautions: Butterbur is considered safe when used as directed. However, it is essential to choose products labeled "PA-free," as some Butterbur products may contain pyrrolizidine alkaloids (PAs), which can harm the liver and cause other adverse effects. Consult with a healthcare provider before using Butterbur, especially if you are pregnant, nursing, or have any underlying health concerns. Some individuals may experience minor gastrointestinal discomfort or skin rashes while using Butterbur. If adverse reactions occur, discontinue use, and consult with a healthcare provider.

Use Butterbur supplements from reputable sources to ensure product quality and safety. Always consult a healthcare provider before starting any new supplement or treatment regimen, especially if you have underlying health concerns or are taking medications.

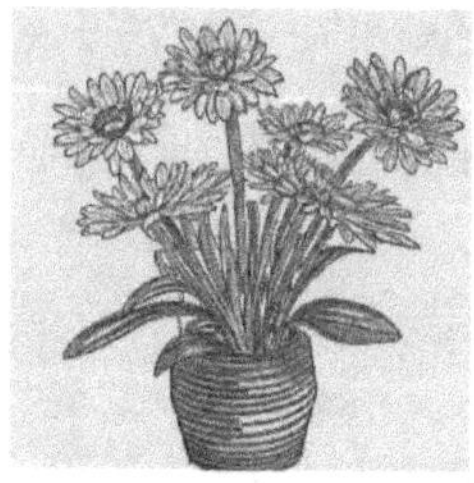

Calendula (Calendula officinalis) is a bright and cheerful flowering plant known for its medicinal and culinary uses. It has a long history of use in traditional herbal medicine and is appreciated for its vibrant orange and yellow blossoms. Here is a detailed overview of its historical use, current medically proven uses, visual identification, growth conditions, care, preparation for medicinal use, and precautions.

Historical Use: Calendula has been used for centuries in traditional medicine, particularly in Europe, for its anti-inflammatory, antimicrobial, and wound-healing properties. It was also used for culinary purposes, such as adding color and flavor to dishes, and as a dye.

Medicinal Properties: Wound Healing: Calendula is commonly used as a topical treatment for minor wounds, burns, and skin irritations. It can promote the healing of minor cuts and abrasions.
Anti-Inflammatory: It is anti-inflammatory and may be used to soothe inflamed skin conditions. Antimicrobial: Calendula has mild antimicrobial properties that can help protect against infection. Skin Conditions: It may be used for specific skin conditions like eczema and psoriasis, although more research is needed.

Visual Identification: Calendula plants can be recognized by the following characteristics: Bright orange or yellow daisy-like flowers with a prominent central disk. Leaves are lance-shaped and green with a slightly hairy texture. The plant typically grows to a height of about 1-2 feet.

Growth Conditions: Calendula is a hardy plant that can be grown in many regions. It prefers well-drained soil and full sun but can tolerate some shade. It is an annual or short-lived perennial.

Care: Plant Calendula seeds in well-drained soil in early spring. Water regularly, but avoid overwatering, as it can lead to root rot.
Deadhead (remove spent flowers) to encourage continuous blooming. Calendula is pest-resistant, making it a suitable choice for organic gardening.

Preparation for Medicinal Use: Calendula is commonly used as topical preparations such as creams, ointments, and salves. To make a basic Calendula salve at home: Harvest Calendula flowers when they are fully open. Dry the flowers by hanging them upside down in a cool, dark, well-ventilated area. Once dried, infuse the dried flowers in a carrier oil (e.g., olive oil) by placing them in a glass jar and covering them with the oil. Seal the jar on a sunny windowsill for about 2-4 weeks. Strain the oil and use it to make a salve by melting it with beeswax. Pour the mixture into small containers and let it cool to solidify.

Precautions:
Calendula is considered safe for external use. However, it may cause skin irritation in some individuals. Perform a patch test before using Calendula products extensively. If you are pregnant, nursing, have allergies, or have underlying health concerns, consult a healthcare provider before using Calendula, especially if you plan to use it internally. Always consult a healthcare provider before using Calendula for medicinal purposes, especially if you have allergies or are dealing with specific skin conditions.

Caprylic acid is a type of saturated fatty acid found in certain foods and used as a dietary supplement. It is a medium-chain triglyceride (MCT) with various potential health benefits. Here is an overview of caprylic acid, its sources, uses, and precautions.

Sources: Caprylic acid is naturally present in the following food sources: Coconut oil is one of the richest dietary sources of caprylic acid. Palm kernel oil: Palm kernel oil also contains caprylic acid. Dairy products: Some dairy products, such as cow's milk, contain tiny amounts of caprylic acid.

Potential Uses: Known for its antimicrobial properties, which can help fight against certain bacteria, fungi, and yeast. It may combat infections caused by Candida yeast and other pathogens. Brain Health: As an MCT, caprylic acid is believed to have potential benefits for brain health. It can provide a quick energy source for the brain and is sometimes used as part of a ketogenic diet for neurological conditions. Weight Management: MCTs, including caprylic acid, have been studied for their potential to support weight management and promote fat burning. Skin Health: Some topical skincare products contain caprylic acid due to its potential benefits for skin health.

Precautions: Dietary Sources: When consumed as part of a normal diet, caprylic acid is considered safe. However, consuming it in moderation is essential as part of a balanced diet. Supplements: If using caprylic acid supplements, following the recommended dosage guidelines is crucial. Excessive consumption of MCTs can lead to digestive issues, including diarrhea and stomach cramps. Allergies: Some individuals may be allergic or sensitive to MCTs, so it is important to be aware of any adverse reactions.

Consult with a healthcare provider before using caprylic acid supplements, especially if you are pregnant, nursing, or have underlying health conditions.

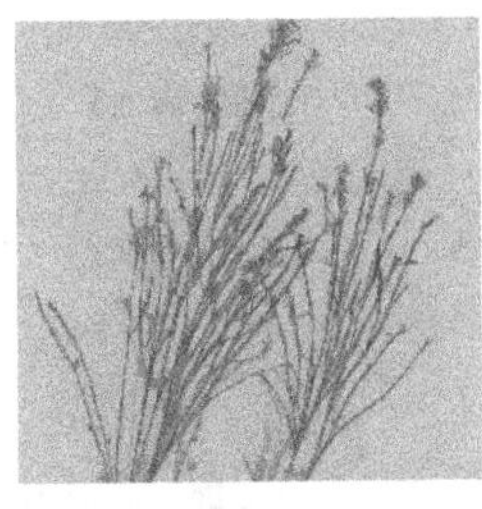 **Caraway (Carum carvi)** is a biennial herb that has been used for centuries in culinary and medicinal applications. It is well-known for its distinctive aroma and flavor, which is often described as warm and slightly sweet. Here is a detailed overview of caraway, including its historical use, current culinary and medicinal uses, visual identification, growth conditions, care, and precautions.

Historical Use: Caraway has a long history of use, dating back to ancient times. It was used by the ancient Egyptians, Greeks, and Romans for various culinary and medicinal purposes. In traditional herbal medicine, caraway was employed to aid digestion and relieve various gastrointestinal issues.

Current Culinary Uses: Caraway seeds are a popular spice in many cuisines and are known for their distinctive flavor. They are commonly used in Breads and Baked Goods: Caraway seeds are often added to bread, rolls, and crackers for their flavor and aroma. Pickles and Sauerkraut: Caraway seeds are a key ingredient in traditional pickle recipes. Cheeses: Some cheeses, such as Havarti and Muenster, are flavored with caraway seeds. Liqueurs: Caraway is used in some liqueurs, such as aquavit and kümmel.

Current Medicinal Uses: Caraway is used in herbal medicine for its digestive benefits, including Digestive Aid. Caraway is believed to help relieve digestive discomfort, such as bloating, gas, and indigestion. Antispasmodic: It is used to reduce stomach cramps and spasms. Appetite Stimulation: Caraway may help stimulate the appetite.

Visual Identification: Caraway plants can be recognized by the following characteristics: Feathery leaves that resemble carrot or parsley leaves. Umbrella-shaped clusters of small white or pink flowers. Small, crescent-shaped (caraway seeds) are produced in the flower heads and used as a spice.

Growth Conditions: Caraway is a biennial plant that prefers well-drained, loamy soil and full sun. It can be grown in various climates but is best suited for temperate regions.

Care: Plant caraway seeds in the spring or fall, spacing them several inches apart. Keep the soil consistently moist but not waterlogged. Support the tall flower stalks, which can become top-heavy and may need staking.

Precautions: Caraway is considered safe when used in culinary amounts. However, some individuals may be sensitive to caraway and experience allergic reactions. If using caraway for medicinal purposes, consult with a healthcare provider, especially if you are pregnant, nursing, or have underlying gastrointestinal conditions.
Caraway is a versatile spice with a long history of culinary and medicinal use. It can add a unique and flavorful twist to various dishes while potentially offering digestive benefits when used in herbal remedies.

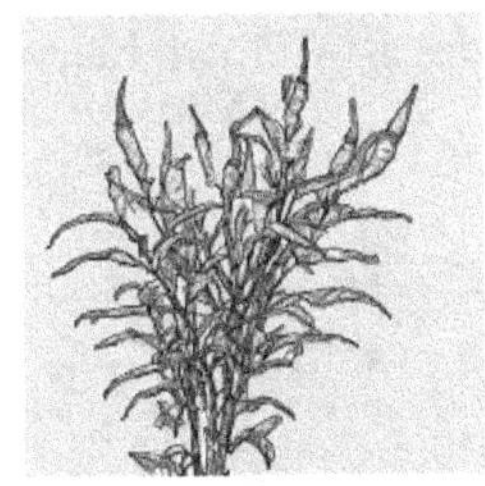 **Cayenne pepper (Capsicum annuum)** is a hot chili pepper variety that is widely known for its pungent and spicy flavor. It is used both in culinary dishes and traditional medicine for its potential health benefits. Here is a detailed overview of cayenne pepper, including its historical use, culinary uses, medicinal properties, visual identification, growth conditions, care, precautions, and potential health benefits.

Historical Use: Cayenne pepper has a long history of use, dating back centuries. Native American tribes' health-related purposes.

Culinary Uses: Cayenne pepper is a popular spice that adds heat and flavor to many dishes, including sauces and condiments. Cayenne is a key ingredient in hot sauces, such as t sauce. Spicy Dishes: It is used in various spicy dishes, such as curries, chili, and salsa. Marinades: Cayenne is used in marinades for meats and poultry. Baking: It can be added to baked goods like bread, muffins, and brownies for a spicy kick.

Medicinal Properties: Cayenne pepper is known for its potential health benefits, including Pain Relief. It may be used topically as a natural pain reliever for arthritis, muscle pain, and nerve pain. Digestive Health: Cayenne can stimulate digestion and help relieve indigestion. Circulatory Health: It is believed to promote healthy circulation and may help support cardiovascular health. Weight Management: Some studies suggest that cayenne may boost metabolism and promote weight loss.

Anti-Inflammatory Properties: Cayenne has anti-inflammatory properties that may benefit certain conditions.

Visual Identification: Cayenne pepper plants can be recognized by the following characteristics: Compact, bushy plants with lance-shaped leaves. Small, elongated chili peppers that are green when unripe and turn red when mature. The level of spiciness varies among cayenne pepper varieties.

Growth Conditions: Cayenne peppers are typically grown as annuals and require well-drained soil and full sun. They can be grown in gardens, containers, or as potted plants.

Care: Plant cayenne pepper seeds or transplants in the spring after the last frost. Provide regular watering, ensuring the soil is consistently moist but not waterlogged. Support the plants with stakes or cages, as they can grow tall and become top-heavy with fruit.

Precautions: Cayenne pepper is spicy and can cause discomfort if consumed excessively. Topical use of cayenne products can lead to skin irritation, especially in individuals with sensitive skin. Consult with a healthcare provider before using cayenne for medicinal purposes, especially if you are pregnant, nursing, or have underlying health conditions. Cayenne pepper is a flavorful and spicy addition to many dishes, it also offers potential health benefits valued in culinary and traditional medicine.

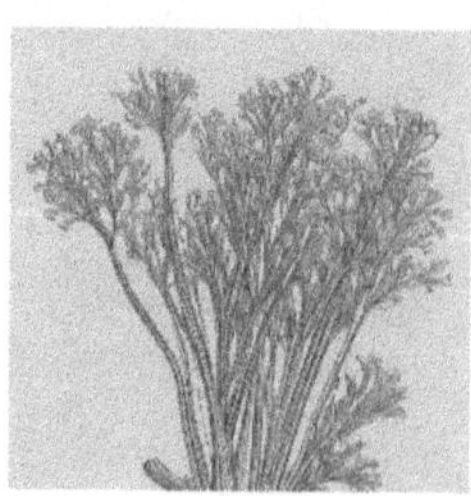

Celery seed (Apium graveolens) is a spice derived from the celery plant's seeds. It is used both in culinary applications and traditional herbal

medicine. Here is a detailed overview of celery seed, including its historical use, culinary uses, medicinal properties, visual identification, growth conditions, care, precautions, and potential health benefits.

Historical Use:have been used for various purposes. In traditional herbal medicine, celery seed has been used for potential health benefits.

Culinary Uses: Celery seed is a spice known for its earthy and slightly bitter flavor. It is used in various culinary applications, including Pickling. Celery seed is commonly used in pickling recipes for its distinctive flavor. Spice Blends: A common ingredient in spice blends like Old Bay seasoning. Salad Dressings: Celery seed is used in some salad dressings to add depth of flavor.
Soups and Stews: It can be added to soups and stews for a hint of celery flavor.

Medicinal Properties: Celery seed has been traditionally used in herbal medicine for its potential health benefits, including Anti-Inflammatory: It is believed to have anti-inflammatory properties and may be used to help manage conditions associated with inflammation. Digestive Health: Celery seed is sometimes used to aid digestion and alleviate gastrointestinal discomfort.
Blood Pressure: Some studies suggest celery seed extract may help lower blood pressure. Antioxidant: Celery seed contains antioxidants that can help protect cells from oxidative stress.

Visual Identification: The celery seed is small, oval, and brown.

It is typically sold as whole seeds and is often ground into a powder for use in recipes.

Growth Conditions: Celery is a biennial plant that is grown for its stalks as well as its seeds. It prefers cool temperatures and well-drained soil. The seeds are typically harvested in the second year when the plant produces flowers and seeds.

Care: Celery plants require consistent moisture and cool growing conditions. Celery seed is harvested from the mature flowers of the celery plant. The seeds are collected when the seed heads have dried and turned brown.

Precautions: While celery seed is considered safe when used in culinary amounts, it may cause an allergic reaction in some individuals.

Consult with a healthcare provider before using celery seed for medicinal purposes, especially if you are pregnant, nursing, or have underlying health conditions.

As with any dietary supplement, moderation is important and should not be used as a sole treatment for medical conditions. Celery seed is a versatile spice with both culinary and potential medicinal uses. It adds a unique flavor to dishes and may offer health benefits when used in herbal remedies, but it should be used in moderation. Always consult with a healthcare provider before using it for specific health concerns.

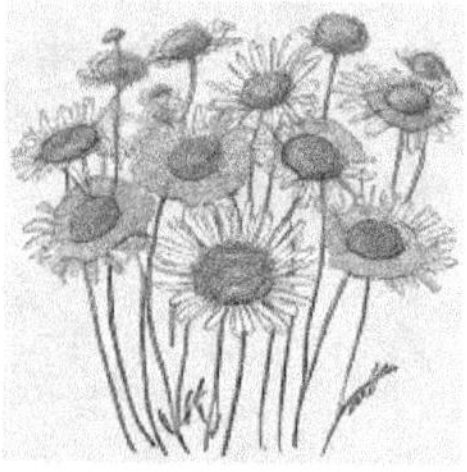

Chamomile (Matricaria chamomilla), also known as German chamomile, is a popular herb known for its numerous culinary, medicinal, and therapeutic uses. It is renowned for its mild,

apple-like aroma and is used in various forms, including teas, essential oils, and topical creams. Here is a detailed overview of chamomile, including its historical use, culinary and medicinal uses, visual identification, growth conditions, care, precautions, and potential health benefits.

Historical Use: Chamomile has a long history of use dating back centuries. It was widely used by ancient civilizations, including the Greeks, Egyptians, and Romans, for its potential medicinal properties. It is often called the "plant's physician" because it was thought to promote nearby plants' health.

Culinary Uses: Chamomile flowers are used in culinary applications, particularly herbal teas. Chamomile tea is known for its mild and soothing flavor. It is often consumed for relaxation and as a sleep aid. The flowers can also be flavored or garnished in salads, desserts, and baked goods.

Medicinal Properties: Chamomile is used in traditional herbal medicine for its potential health benefits, including relaxation and sleep. Chamomile tea is consumed for its calming and sleep-inducing properties. Digestive Health: It is used to alleviate digestive discomfort, such as indigestion, gas, and bloating. Anti-Inflammatory: Chamomile has anti-inflammatory properties that may be useful for skin conditions and wound healing. Skin Care: Chamomile is a common ingredient in skincare products, including creams, lotions, and essential oils, for its soothing effect on the skin. Anti-Anxiety: It may help reduce symptoms of anxiety and stress.

Visual Identification: Chamomile plants can be recognized by the following characteristics: Fine, feathery leaves. Small, daisy-like flowers with white petals and a yellow center. A pleasant, apple-like fragrance when crushed.

Growth Conditions: Chamomile is a low-growing annual herb that prefers well-drained, sandy soil and full sun. It is easy to grow and can be cultivated in gardens or containers.

Care: Plant chamomile seeds in early spring or early autumn. Keep the soil consistently moist but not waterlogged. Harvest the flowers for culinary and medicinal purposes when they are fully open.

Precautions: While chamomile is considered safe when used in moderate amounts, some individuals may be sensitive or allergic to it. Allergic reactions are rare but can occur. If you are allergic to plants in the Asteraceae family (such as ragweed, marigolds, or daisies), you may be more likely to be allergic to chamomile. Consult with a healthcare provider before using chamomile for medicinal purposes, especially if you are pregnant, nursing, or have underlying health conditions. Chamomile is a versatile herb with a gentle, soothing nature and a wide range of potential health benefits. It is a beloved ingredient in the world of herbal teas and skin care products and is appreciated for its calming and therapeutic properties.

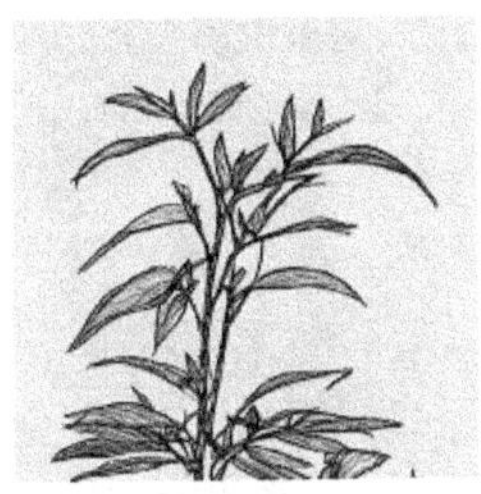

Chasteberry also known as Vitex agnus-castus or simply Vitex, is a popular herb with a history of traditional use for various health concerns, particularly in women's health. It is native to the Mediterranean region and has been used for centuries in herbal medicine.

Historical Use: Chasteberry has a long history of use, dating back to ancient times. It was traditionally used in Greek and Roman medicine to address various women's health issues. The name "chasteberry" comes from the belief that it had the power to curb sexual desire. However, it is not used for that purpose today.

Medicinal Properties: Chasteberry is primarily used for its potential effects on women's health, including Hormone Regulation. It is often used to help regulate menstrual cycles and relieve symptoms associated with premenstrual syndrome (PMS) and menopause. Fertility Support: Some women use chasteberry to improve fertility by regulating ovulation and addressing hormonal imbalances. Breast Tenderness: Chasteberry may help alleviate breast tenderness associated with the menstrual cycle. Acne and Skin Health: It is sometimes used to manage hormonal acne.

Visual Identification: Chasteberry plants can be recognized by the following characteristics: A small, deciduous shrub or tree with lance-shaped leaves. Clusters of violet-blue flowers with a distinctive fragrance. The plant produces small, hard, deep brown to black fruits, which are the "chasteberry" seeds.

Growth Conditions: Chasteberry is native to Mediterranean regions but can be cultivated in various climates. It prefers well-drained soil and full sun to partial shade.

Care: Plant chasteberry in well-drained soil and ensure regular watering during its establishment phase. The plant requires minimal pruning and maintenance once it has established itself.

Precautions: Chasteberry is considered safe for most individuals when used as directed. It may take several months of consistent use for the full effects to be realized. Some individuals may experience mild gastrointestinal discomfort or headaches. Consult with a healthcare provider before using chasteberry, especially if you are pregnant, nursing, have underlying health conditions, or are taking medications.

Chasteberry is a versatile herb with a focus on women's health. It is valued for its potential to regulate hormonal imbalances and relieve various menstrual and menopausal symptoms. Always consult a healthcare provider before using chasteberry for specific health concerns, especially if you have underlying health conditions, are pregnant, or are nursing.

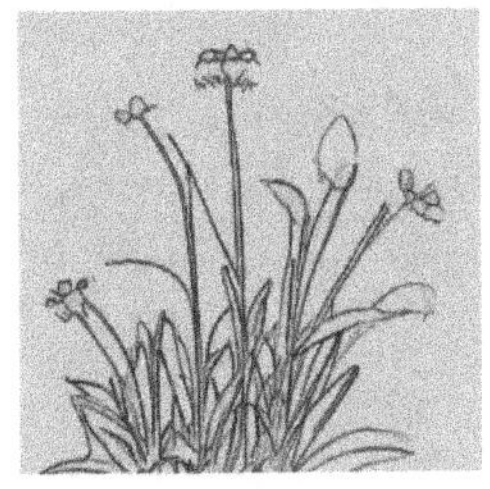

Chickweed (Stellaria media) is a common and widely distributed herbaceous plant that is often considered a weed. However, it has a long history of use in traditional herbal medicine and can also be a nutritious edible green. Here is a detailed overview of chickweed, including its historical use, culinary uses, medicinal properties, visual identification, growth conditions, care, precautions, and potential health benefits.

Historical Use: Chickweed has a history of use in traditional herbal medicine, dating back centuries. It was traditionally employed for various health-related purposes, including treating skin conditions and digestive discomfort.

Culinary Uses: Chickweed is edible and can be used in culinary applications, including Salads. It can be added to salads for its mild, slightly nutty flavor. Pesto: Chickweed can be used as a substitute for basil in pesto recipes. Stir-Fries: It can be lightly sautéed and included in stir-fry dishes. Herbal Teas: Some people make herbal teas from chickweed, although it is not as common as its culinary use.

Medicinal Properties: Chickweed is used in herbal medicine for its potential health benefits, including skin health. It is believed to soothe skin conditions such as eczema, psoriasis, and minor burns. Anti-Inflammatory: Chickweed has anti-inflammatory properties that may help alleviate inflammation. Digestive Health: It soothes digestive discomfort, such as indigestion and gastritis.

Visual Identification: Chickweed plants can be recognized by the following characteristics: Small, low-growing herbaceous plants with pairs of small, oval-shaped leaves. Tiny, star-shaped white flowers with five petals. The stems are often sprawling and can form dense mats.

Growth Conditions: Chickweed is a hardy plant found in various habitats, including gardens, lawns, and open fields. It thrives in cool, moist environments.

Care: Chickweed is often considered a weed and can thrive in various soil types. It does not require specific care or maintenance in cultivated gardens, as it tends to self-sow and spread easily.

Precautions: Chickweed is considered safe when used as a food or for topical applications. However, it should be identified confidently to avoid potentially toxic look-alike plants. As with any herbal remedy, consult a healthcare provider before using chickweed for specific health concerns, especially if you have underlying health conditions or are taking medications. When foraging for chickweed, harvest it from clean, pesticide-free areas. Chickweed is a versatile herb that can be used both in culinary applications and for potential medicinal benefits. As with any herb or wild plant, it is essential to properly identify it and consult with a healthcare provider before using it for medicinal purposes, especially if you have allergies or underlying health conditions.

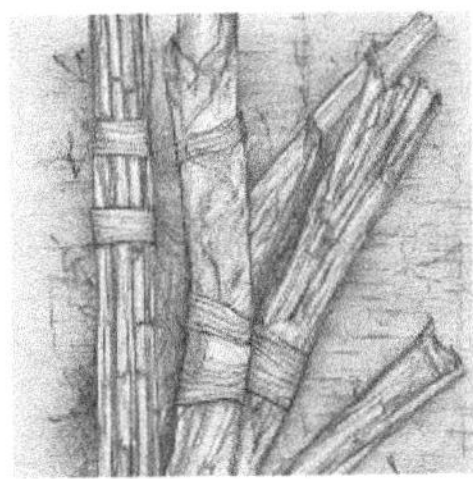

Cinnamon is a highly aromatic spice from the bark of trees belonging to the Cinnamomum family. It is not only known for its delightful flavor but also for its potential health benefits. Here is an overview of cinnamon, including its historical use, medicinal uses, visual identification, growth conditions, preparation, and health benefits:

Historical Use: Cinnamon has a rich history of use dating back to ancient civilizations. It was highly regarded in traditional medicine systems and was prized for its aroma and flavor. Cinnamon has been used for various purposes, including culinary, medicinal, and perfumery.

Medicinal Uses: Cinnamon has been used for centuries in traditional medicine for its potential health benefits. Some of its commonly known medicinal uses include Anti-Inflammatory Properties: Cinnamon is believed to have anti-inflammatory effects, which may help reduce inflammation and inflammation-related conditions. Antioxidant Activity: Cinnamon is rich in antioxidants that help combat oxidative stress and protect the body from free radicals. Blood Sugar Management: Some studies suggest that cinnamon may help regulate blood sugar levels and improve insulin sensitivity, benefiting people with diabetes or those at risk.

Heart Health: Cinnamon may support heart health by reducing blood pressure and lowering bad cholesterol levels. Anti-Microbial Effects: Cinnamon contains compounds with antimicrobial properties, which may help fight various pathogens, including bacteria and fungi.

Visual Identification: Cinnamon is derived from the bark of the Cinnamomum tree. Here are some characteristics to help identify cinnamon: Cinnamon bark is brown with a fragrant aroma.

The outer bark is hard and rough, while the inner bark is softer and can be peeled away in thin strips or rolled into Sticks. Cinnamon sticks are often used in cooking and have a woody texture and a sweet, warm flavor. Cinnamon powder is made from ground cinnamon sticks and has a fine, brownish appearance.

Growth Conditions: Cinnamon is typically grown in tropical and subtropical regions. Some factors to consider when cultivating cinnamon include Geographical Area: Cinnamon is primarily grown in countries like Sri Lanka, India, Indonesia, and Vietnam. Cultivation: It is cultivated as a tree, and the bark is harvested for culinary and medicinal use. Climate: Cinnamon trees thrive in warm, humid climates with well-distributed rainfall. Soil: The soil should be well-draining, loamy, and slightly acidic, with a pH level between 6.0 and 7.0.

Preparation and Health Benefits: Cinnamon can be used in various forms to derive its potential health benefits: Ground Cinnamon: Ground cinnamon can be added to a wide range of recipes, such as baked goods, oatmeal, and beverages, to impart its distinctive flavor and health benefits. [OBJ] Cinnamon Sticks: Cinnamon sticks are often used to infuse flavors in hot beverages like tea and mulled wine. They can also be used for culinary and decorative purposes.

Cinnamon Oil: Cinnamon essential oil is used for aromatherapy, massage, and certain medicinal purposes. It is important to dilute cinnamon oil before using it topically, and it should not be ingested without proper guidance. It is important to note that while cinnamon is recognized as safe and offers various health benefits, its use should be moderate, and it may not be suitable for everyone. Cinnamon supplements and large quantities of cassia cinnamon should be used cautiously, especially by people with liver conditions, allergies, or other medical concerns.

It is advisable to consult with a healthcare provider or herbalist to determine the most appropriate form and dosage for your individual needs.

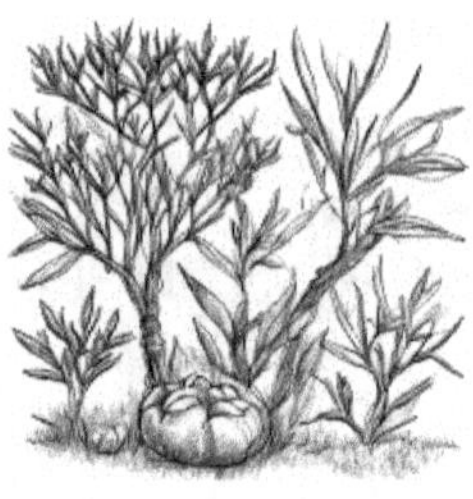

Clove, derived from the dried flower buds of the Syzygium aromaticum tree, is a spice known for its warm, sweet, and aromatic flavor. It has a rich history of medicinal use and is a versatile ingredient in both culinary and traditional medicine applications. Here is an overview of clove, including its historical use, medicinal uses, visual identification, growth conditions, preparation, and potential health benefits:

Historical Use: Clove has a long history of use dating back thousands of years. It was highly regarded in traditional medicine systems, particularly Ayurvedic and traditional Chinese medicine. Clove has been used for its aromatic qualities, culinary applications, and potential medicinal benefits.

Medicinal Uses: Clove is valued for its potential health benefits and has been used in traditional medicine for various purposes. Some of its commonly known medicinal uses include Pain Relief: Clove oil and clove-derived compounds, such as eugenol, have analgesic properties and have been used to relieve dental pain, sore throats, and headaches. Antioxidant Properties: Clove is rich in antioxidants, which help combat oxidative stress and free radicals in the body. Antibacterial and Antifungal Effects: Clove has shown antibacterial and antifungal properties and has been used to treat infections and oral health issues. Anti-Inflammatory Effects: Eugenol, a major component of clove, has anti-inflammatory properties and may help reduce inflammation.
Digestive Aid: Clove has been used to aid digestion and relieve gastrointestinal discomfort. Respiratory Health: It relieves coughs, colds, and respiratory issues. Dental Health: Clove is used in oral care products due to its potential to combat bad breath, gum disease, and dental infections.

Visual Identification: Clove is derived from the dried flower buds of the clove tree and has the following characteristics: Dried cloves are small, deep brown, hard, and nail shaped. The taste and aroma of clove are warm, sweet, and aromatic. Clove powder is made by grinding dried cloves into a fine, deep brown powder.

Growth Conditions: Clove trees are native to the Maluku Islands in Indonesia but are also cultivated in other tropical regions. Here are some factors to consider when growing clove: Geographical Area: Clove is primarily grown in countries such as Indonesia, Madagascar, and Sri Lanka. Cultivation: Clove trees are grown from seeds or cuttings and require well-drained soil. Climate: Clove trees thrive in tropical climates with abundant rainfall and moderate humidity. Soil: The soil should be well-drained and slightly acidic, with a pH level between 6.0 and 6.5.

Preparation and Health Benefits: Cloves can be used in various forms to derive their potential health benefits. Whole Cloves: Whole cloves are used for culinary purposes and can be added to recipes for flavor and aroma. They can also be used to infuse hot beverages like tea and mulled wine. Ground Clove: Ground clove is a versatile spice in sweet and savory dishes. It can be added to desserts, curries, soups, and spice blends. Clove Oil: Clove essential oil is used in aromatherapy, massage, and certain medicinal applications. It should be used cautiously, and dilution is recommended for topical use. Clove is considered safe when used in moderate amounts as a spice or flavoring agent in cooking. However, undiluted clove oil can be potent and should only be ingested or applied topically with proper guidance.

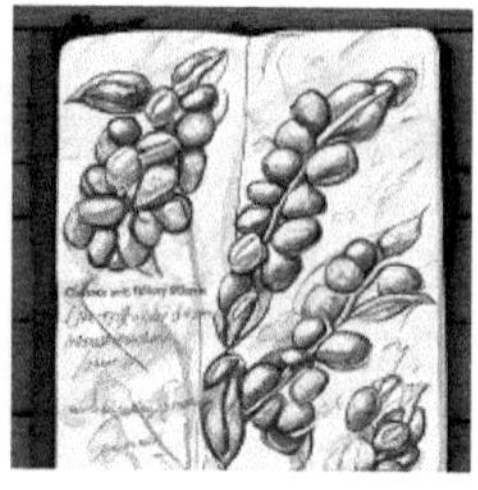

Coffee (Coffea) is a popular and widely consumed beverage made from the seeds of coffee plants. It is known for its stimulating effects and rich, complex flavors. Coffee is one of the most traded and consumed beverages in the world. Here is a detailed overview of coffee, including its historical use, varieties, cultivation, preparation, potential health benefits, and precautions.

Historical Use: Coffee has a long and storied history that dates back to ancient times. It is believed to have been first consumed in the region that is now Ethiopia. Coffee houses, known as "qahveh khaneh," became popular in the Middle East in the 16th century and later spread to Europe. Coffee's energizing effects made it a favorite beverage among various cultures.

Varieties: There are several species of coffee, but the most cultivated for consumption are Coffea arabica (Arabica coffee) and Coffea canephora (Robusta coffee). Arabica coffee is known for its smooth, mild flavor, while Robusta coffee has a stronger, more bitter taste.

Cultivation: Coffee is grown in various world regions, primarily in tropical and subtropical climates. The cultivation of coffee involves several stages, including growing, harvesting, processing, and roasting. Coffee is typically grown on large plantations or small family farms.

Preparation: Coffee can be prepared in numerous ways, with the most common method being brewing with hot water. Here are a few popular coffee preparation methods: Drip Coffee: Ground coffee is placed in a filter, and hot water drips through it into a pot or carafe. Espresso: Finely ground coffee is packed into a portafilter, and hot water is forced through it, producing a concentrated coffee shot. French Press: Coarsely ground coffee is steeped in hot water, and a metal or mesh plunger separates the grounds. AeroPress: A portable device that uses air pressure to brew a single cup of coffee. Pour-Over: Hot water is manually poured over coffee grounds in a filter, allowing the liquid to flow through and extract the coffee.

Potential Health Benefits: Coffee has been the subject of extensive research, and some potential health benefits include Caffeine's Stimulating Effects: Coffee can provide increased alertness and concentration due to its caffeine content. Antioxidants: Coffee is a rich source of antioxidants, which may help protect cells from oxidative damage. Reduced Risk of Certain Diseases: Some studies suggest that coffee consumption is associated with a lower risk of certain diseases, including Parkinson's disease, type 2 diabetes, and certain types of cancer. Mood Enhancement: Coffee can boost mood and reduce the risk of depression.

Precautions:
While moderate coffee consumption is safe for most people, excessive coffee intake can lead to side effects such as restlessness, insomnia, and increased heart rate. Caffeine sensitivity varies among individuals, so knowing your tolerance is important. Pregnant individuals should limit their caffeine intake, and those with certain medical conditions should consult a healthcare provider about coffee consumption.

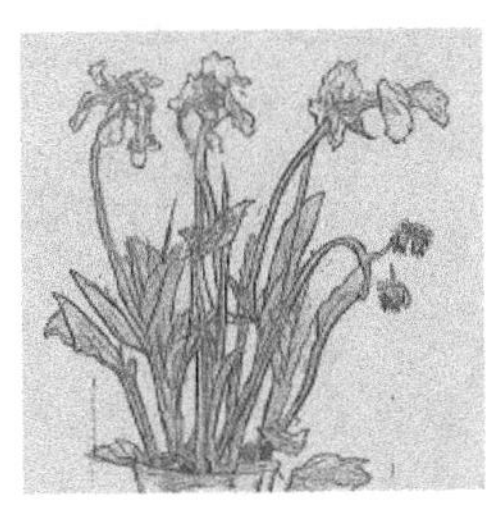

Comfrey (Symphytum officinale) is a perennial herb used for centuries in traditional herbal medicine for

291

its potential medicinal benefits. It is known for its robust growth and has a variety of uses, although its use has raised safety concerns in recent years due to the presence of potentially harmful compounds. Here is a detailed overview of comfrey, including its historical use, medicinal properties, visual identification, growth conditions, care, precautions, and potential health benefits.

Historical Use:
Comfrey has a long history of use in traditional herbal medicine, particularly in Europe. It was used for a wide range of purposes, including wound healing, soothing skin conditions, and addressing digestive discomfort.

Medicinal Properties: Comfrey is traditionally used for its potential health benefits, including wound healing. It has been used topically to promote wound healing and reduce inflammation. Joint and Muscle Pain: Comfrey has been used in topical applications, such as ointments, for relieving joint and muscle pain. Anti-Inflammatory: Some believe comfrey has anti-inflammatory properties that may help with certain conditions.

Visual Identification: Comfrey plants can be recognized by the following characteristics: Large, hairy leaves that are often dark green and lance shaped. Clusters of small, bell-shaped flowers can be an assortment of colors, including white, blue, or purple. Thick, robust stems that can reach several feet in height.

Growth Conditions: Comfrey is a hardy plant that can be grown in various soil types and climates. It prefers well-drained soil and partial to full sun.

Care: Comfrey can be propagated by root cuttings, divisions, or seeds. Once established, the plant requires little care but can be invasive if not controlled. Regular pruning can help manage its growth and prevent it from spreading excessively.

Precautions: Comfrey contains pyrrolizidine alkaloids, which are potentially toxic compounds. These alkaloids can harm the liver and cause serious health issues when consumed or applied topically over extended periods. Due to the presence of these alkaloids, comfrey is not recommended for internal use, and its external use should be limited to short periods and under the guidance of a healthcare provider. Pregnant or nursing individuals, children, and individuals with liver conditions should avoid comfrey use. While comfrey has a history of traditional use, its potential toxicity has led to concerns about its safety. It is essential to be cautious when using comfrey, especially when considering its internal use. Consult with a healthcare provider before using comfrey for medicinal purposes and avoid using it if you are in a high-risk category, such as pregnant or nursing.

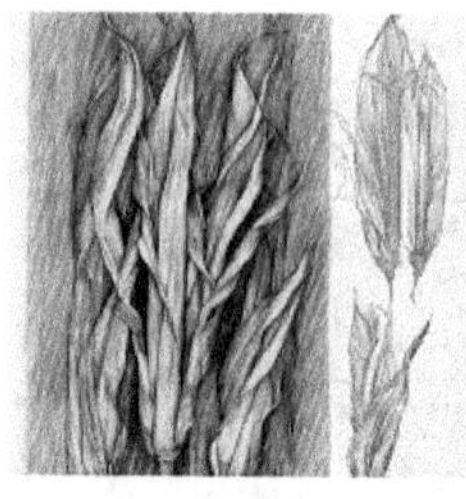

Corn silk, also known as maize silk, refers to the long, thread-like fibers that extend from the tops of the ears of corn (maize). While it is often discarded and not consumed as part of the corn cob, corn silk has a history of traditional use for its potential health benefits. Here is an overview of corn silk, including its historical use, medicinal uses, visual identification, growth conditions, preparation, and potential health benefits.

Historical Use: Corn silk has a long history of use in traditional medicine systems, particularly among Indigenous cultures in North and Central America. Native American tribes and traditional herbalists used it for various health purposes.

Medicinal Uses: Corn silk is valued for its potential health benefits and has been used in traditional medicine for various purposes. Some of its commonly known medicinal uses include Diuretic Properties: Corn silk is known for its diuretic effect, which means it may promote urine production and help flush excess water and waste from the body. It has been used to address water retention, edema, and urinary tract.

Health issues. Bladder and Kidney Support: Corn silk has been used to soothe and support the urinary tract, potentially benefiting those with urinary discomfort or mild urinary tract issues.
Prostate Health: Some herbal traditions suggest that corn silk may be helpful for prostate health, though scientific evidence supporting this is limited. Antioxidant Activity: Corn silk contains antioxidants, which can help combat oxidative stress in the body and promote overall health. Antioxidant Activity: Corn

silk contains antioxidants, which can help combat oxidative stress in the body and promote overall health.

Visual Identification: Corn silk refers to the long, silky, hair-like threads that emerge from the tips of corn ears (cobs) before the corn kernels fully develop. These fine, golden, or pale threads can be easily identified by their appearance and are typically removed when preparing corn for consumption.

Growth Conditions: Corn is a warm-season, annual crop grown for its edible kernels. Here are some factors to consider when growing corn: Geographical Area: Corn is widely cultivated in many countries, with various cultivars adapted to different climates. Cultivation: Corn is grown from seeds (kernels) and requires adequate spacing and well-drained soil. Climate: Corn thrives in warm, sunny conditions and requires frost-free weather during the growing season. Soil: It prefers fertile, well-draining soil with a slightly acidic to neutral pH.

Preparation and Health Benefits: Corn silk can be used in different forms to derive potential health benefits. Tea: Corn silk can be dried and used to make corn silk tea. To prepare corn silk tea, simply steep the dried silk in hot water, strain it, and drink it as a beverage. It is often enjoyed for its diuretic properties, potentially aiding in the reduction of water retention. Supplements: Corn silk is available in supplement form, including capsules and extracts. These supplements are typically taken as directed by a healthcare provider or herbalist. If you have any underlying health conditions or are taking medications, consult with a healthcare provider before incorporating corn silk into your wellness routine. Additionally, it is advisable to obtain corn silk from a reputable supplier.

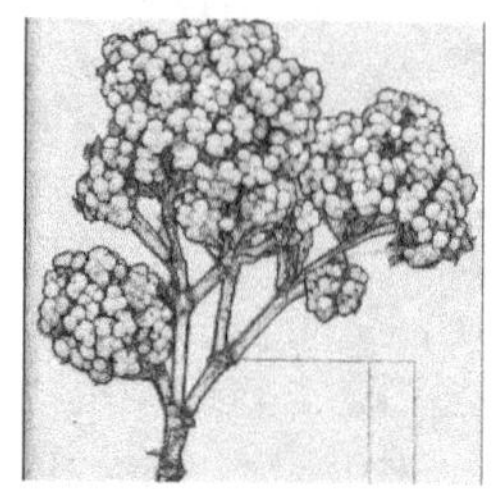

Cramp bark (Viburnum opulus) is a medicinal plant that has been used for centuries in traditional herbal medicine, particularly in Europe and North America. It is known for its potential to alleviate muscle cramps, pain, and discomfort, especially in the context of women's health. Here is a detailed overview of cramp bark, including its historical use, medicinal properties, visual identification, growth conditions, care, precautions, and potential health benefits.

Historical Use: Cramp bark has a long history of use, dating back to Indigenous cultures in North America and Europe. It was traditionally used to address various health concerns, including muscle cramps, menstrual pain, and pregnancy-related discomfort.

Medicinal Properties: Cramp bark is traditionally used for its potential health benefits, including Muscle Relaxant. It is known for its muscle-relaxing properties, making it useful for relieving muscle cramps and spasms. Menstrual Pain: Cramp bark often alleviates menstrual cramps and discomfort. Uterine Health: It is believed to promote uterine health and may be used during pregnancy and childbirth. Anti-Inflammatory: Cramp bark has anti-inflammatory properties that may benefit certain conditions.

Visual Identification: Cramp bark plants can be recognized by the following characteristics: Deciduous shrubs with opposite, serrated leaves. Clusters of white or pinkish flowers with a central flat disc. small, red, or orange berries in the fall that resemble cranberries.

Growth Conditions: Cramp bark is native to North America and Europe. It can be grown in various soil types and is typically found in wooded or forested areas.

Care: Cramp bark can be propagated from seeds, cuttings, or divisions. It requires well-drained soil and is typically minimal maintenance once established.

Precautions: While cramp bark is considered safe when used as directed, it should be used under the guidance of a qualified herbalist or healthcare provider. Pregnant individuals should consult with a healthcare provider before using cramp bark, as its use during pregnancy should be carefully monitored. Some individuals may be allergic to cramp bark or may experience adverse reactions.

Cramp bark is a versatile herb traditionally used for its muscle-relaxing and pain-relieving properties, particularly in women's health. While it is considered safe when used correctly, it is essential to consult with a qualified herbalist or healthcare provider before using it for specific health concerns, especially during pregnancy or if you have allergies or underlying health conditions.

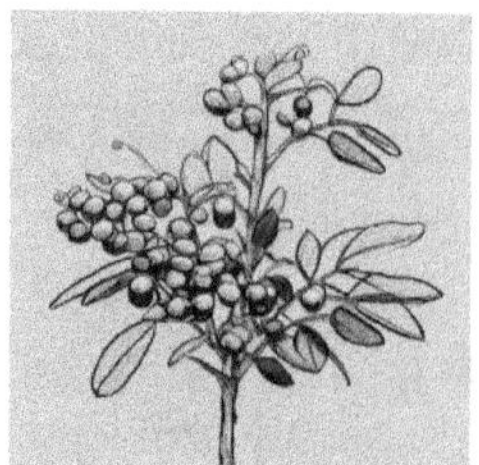**Cranberry (Vaccinium macrocarpon)** is a small, red berry that is native to North America and is known for its tart and slightly sweet flavor. It has a variety of culinary uses and is also associated with several potential health benefits. Here is a detailed overview of cranberries, including their historical use, culinary uses, medicinal properties, visual identification, growth conditions, care, precautions, and potential health benefits:

Historical Use: Cranberries have a long history of use among Native American tribes, who used them as a food source and for their potential medicinal properties. They were introduced to European settlers and have since become a popular fruit in various forms.

Culinary Uses: Cranberries are used in multiple culinary applications, including Sauces. Cranberry sauce is a common accompaniment to roast turkey and other holiday dishes. Baking: Dried or fresh cranberries can be added to muffins, bread, and desserts. Beverages: Cranberry juice is popular, and cranberries are used in cocktails and smoothies. Preserves: Cranberry preserves, and jellies are enjoyed with bread and cheese.

Medicinal Properties: Cranberries have several potential health benefits, including Urinary Tract Health. Cranberries are known for their role in preventing and managing urinary tract infections (UTIs). They contain compounds that may help prevent bacteria from adhering to the urinary tract lining. Antioxidant Properties: Cranberries are rich in antioxidants, which can help protect cells from oxidative damage. Heart Health: Some studies suggest that regular consumption of cranberries may positively impact heart health.

Digestive Health: Cranberries are a useful source of dietary fiber, aiding digestive health.

Visual Identification: Cranberry plants can be recognized by the following characteristics: Low, trailing evergreen shrubs with small, leathery leaves. Delicate pink flowers that develop into small, red berries. Berries are round, small, and typically deep red when ripe.

Growth Conditions: Cranberry plants are grown in wet, acidic, and peat-rich soils. They are often cultivated in bogs and marshes.

Care: Commercial cranberry cultivation involves flooding the fields to facilitate harvesting, as cranberries float when ripe. For home gardeners, cranberry plants can be grown in containers with suitable soil conditions and regular moisture.

Precautions: While cranberries are safe for most people when consumed in moderation, some individuals may be sensitive to them. Cranberry products with added sugar can be high in calories, so it is important to be mindful of sugar intake. Cranberry supplements or large quantities of cranberry juice should be used cautiously, especially by individuals taking blood-thinning medications.

Cranberries are a versatile fruit with both culinary and potential health benefits. They are most famous for their role in supporting urinary tract health and preventing UTIs.

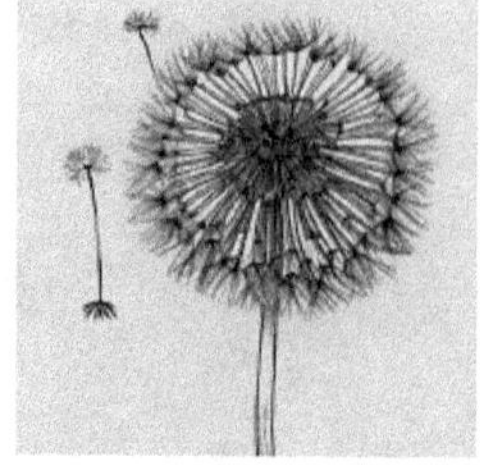

Dandelion (Taraxacum officinale) is a common and widely recognized weed that has a long history of use in both culinary and traditional herbal medicine. It is known for its distinctive yellow flowers and the white, fluffy seed heads that children often blow on to make a wish. Here is a detailed overview of dandelion, including its historical use, culinary uses, medicinal properties, visual identification, growth conditions, care, precautions, and potential health benefits.

Historical Use: Dandelion has been used for centuries in traditional herbal medicine in various cultures worldwide. It has a history of being valued for its potential medicinal properties.

Culinary Uses: Dandelion is edible, and its leaves, flowers, and roots can be used in culinary applications, including Dandelion Greens. Young dandelion leaves can be used in salads and cooked as greens. They have a slightly bitter taste. Dandelion Flowers: The bright yellow flowers can make dandelion wine, syrups, and jellies. Dandelion Roots: The roasted roots can be used as a coffee substitute or as an addition to herbal teas.

Medicinal Properties: Dandelion is used in traditional herbal medicine for its potential health benefits, including digestive health: It is believed to support healthy digestion and may be used for digestive discomfort. Liver Health: Dandelion is often used to promote liver health and detoxification. Diuretic Effects: Dandelion has mild diuretic properties and may be used to increase urine flow. Antioxidant Properties: It contains antioxidants that can help protect cells from oxidative stress.

Visual Identification: Dandelion plants can be recognized by the following characteristics: Rosette of deeply toothed lance-shaped leaves. Bright yellow composite flowers with a central disk and ray petals. White, fluffy seed heads that develop after the flowers go to seed.

Growth Conditions: Dandelions thrive in various environments, including lawns, gardens, fields, and roadsides. They are adaptable and can grow in various soil types and conditions.

Care: Dandelions require little care, as they are hardy and invasive. For culinary use, harvesting them from clean, pesticide-free areas is essential to avoid contamination.

If you are pregnant, nursing, have underlying health conditions, or are taking medications, consult a healthcare provider before using dandelion for medicinal purposes.

Dandelion is a versatile and readily available herb that can be used in culinary applications and for potential health benefits. It is celebrated for its potential digestive, liver, and detoxification support. Always consult a healthcare provider before using dandelion for specific health concerns, especially if you have allergies or underlying health conditions.

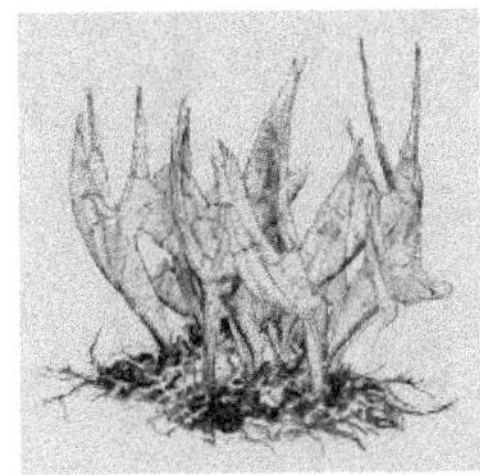

Devil's claw (Harpagophytum procumbens) is a plant native to the Kalahari Desert in southern Africa. It is known for its distinctive hooked fruit, which gives the plant its common name. Devil's claw has a history of use in traditional African medicine and has gained recognition worldwide for its potential health benefits. Here is a detailed overview of devil's claw, including its historical use, medicinal properties, visual identification, growth conditions, care, precautions, and potential health benefits.

Historical Use: Devil's claw has a long history of use among Indigenous peoples of southern Africa. It was traditionally used to address various health concerns, including pain and inflammation.

Medicinal Properties: Devil's claw is known for its potential health benefits, particularly related to pain and inflammation, including
Pain Relief. It is used to alleviate several types of pain, including joint, muscle, and back pain. Anti-Inflammatory: Devil's claw is believed to have anti-inflammatory properties, which can help reduce inflammation and pain.

Digestive Health: It may promote digestive health and alleviate symptoms like heartburn and indigestion. Arthritis: Devil's claw is often used as a natural remedy for osteoarthritis and rheumatoid arthritis.

Visual Identification: Devil's claw plants can be recognized by the following characteristics: Low-growing, perennial herbs with palmate leaves. Reddish-purple, tubular flowers. Hooked, woody fruits, the plant its name.

Growth Conditions: Devil's claw is native to arid and semi-arid regions of southern Africa. It thrives in sandy, well-drained soils and is adapted to hot, dry climates.

Care: Devil's claw can be propagated from seeds or by dividing the rhizomes. It requires minimal maintenance once established and is minimal maintenance.

Precautions: Devil's claw is considered safe when used as directed, although some individuals may experience mild gastrointestinal discomfort. It may interact with certain medications, particularly anticoagulants, and should be used cautiously by individuals taking such medications. Consult with a healthcare provider before using Devil's Claw for specific health concerns, especially if you have underlying health conditions or are taking medications.

Devil's Claw is a unique herbal remedy that has gained recognition for its potential to alleviate pain and inflammation, particularly in the context of arthritis and joint health. It should be used under the guidance of a healthcare provider, especially if you are taking medications or have underlying health conditions. Always seek professional advice before using devil's claw as a natural remedy.

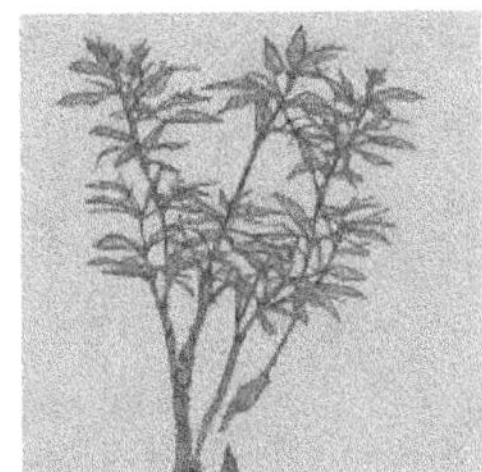 **Dong quai (Angelica sinensis)**, also known as "female ginseng," is a popular herb in traditional Chinese medicine. It has been used for centuries for its potential medicinal benefits, particularly in women's health. Here is a detailed overview of dong quai, including its historical use, medicinal properties, visual identification, growth conditions, care, precautions, and potential health benefits.

Historical Use: Dong quai has a long history of use in traditional Chinese medicine. It is often called the "female ginseng" due to its traditional use for women's health concerns. It has been used to address a wide range of issues, including menstrual problems menopausal symptoms, and as a general tonic.

Medicinal Properties: Dong quai is traditionally used for potential health benefits, including Women's Health. It is commonly used to regulate menstrual cycles, alleviate menstrual cramps, and address menopausal symptoms. Blood Health: Dong quai may have blood-thinning properties and can help improve circulation.
Pain Relief: It is used for pain relief, including headaches and joint pain. Immune System Support: Some traditional uses include immune system support and general health.

Visual Identification: Dong quai plants can be recognized by the following characteristics: tall, slender plants with hollow, purplish stems. Clusters of small white flowers. Triangular, pinnate leaves with serrated edges.

Growth Conditions: Dong quai is native to China and other parts of Asia. It prefers temperate climates and well-drained, fertile soil. It is a biennial plant, meaning it has a two-year life cycle.

Care: Dong quai can be grown from seeds or root cuttings. It requires well-drained soil and full to partial sun. The roots are typically harvested in the fall of the first year or spring of the second year.

Precautions: Dong quai is considered safe when used as directed but should be used under the guidance of a qualified herbalist or healthcare provider.

It may interact with certain medications, particularly blood-thinning drugs, and should be used cautiously by individuals taking such medications. Consult with a healthcare provider before using dong quai for specific health concerns, especially if you are pregnant, nursing, have underlying health conditions, or are taking medications.

Dong quai is a valuable herb in traditional Chinese medicine, particularly for women's health concerns and overall well-being. It should be used with caution and under the guidance of a qualified herbalist or healthcare provider, especially if you are taking medications or have underlying health conditions. Always seek professional advice before using dong quai as a natural remedy.

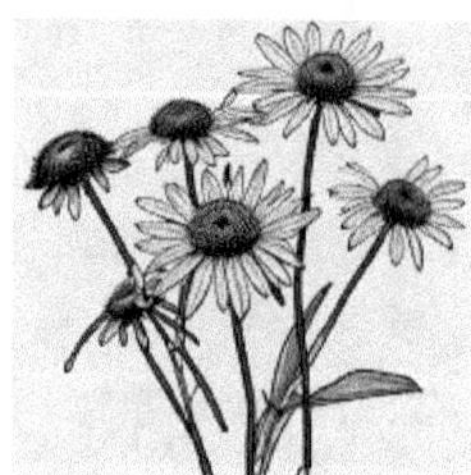

Echinacea (Echinacea purpurea) is a widely recognized herb with a long history of use, particularly among Native American tribes. It is known for its potential medicinal properties and is commonly used to support the immune system and alleviate symptoms of the common cold and other respiratory infections. Here is a detailed overview of echinacea, including its historical use, medicinal properties, visual identification, growth conditions, care, precautions, and potential health benefits.

Historical Use: Echinacea has a history of use among Native American tribes, particularly the Plains Indians, who used it as a traditional herbal remedy for various ailments. It gained popularity in Western herbal medicine in the 19th century.

Medicinal Properties: Echinacea is traditionally used for its potential health benefits, including Immune System Support. It is widely used to support the immune system, particularly during cold and flu seasons. Respiratory Health: Echinacea may help alleviate symptoms of respiratory infections and coughs. Anti-Inflammatory: It is believed to have anti-inflammatory properties, which can help reduce inflammation and pain. Wound Healing: Echinacea is used topically to support wound healing and skin health.

Visual Identification: Echinacea plants can be recognized by the following characteristics: Perennial herb with distinctive daisy-like flowers. Purple, pink, or white petals surrounding a central, raised cone. Coarsely toothed leaves with a rough texture.

Growth Conditions: Echinacea is native to North America and is found in various regions. It thrives in well-drained soil and is typically found in open prairies and fields.

Care: Echinacea can be grown from seeds or root divisions. It requires full sun and well-drained soil. Regular deadheading (removing spent flowers) can encourage more blooms.

Precautions: Echinacea is considered safe for short-term use when used as directed, but it should not be used continuously for extended periods. Some individuals may experience mild gastrointestinal discomfort or allergic reactions. It may interact with certain medications, particularly immunosuppressive drugs, and should be used with caution by individuals taking such medications. Consult with a healthcare provider before using echinacea for specific health concerns, especially if you have underlying health conditions or are taking medications.

Echinacea is a popular herbal remedy, particularly for its potential to support the immune system and alleviate symptoms of respiratory infections. It should be used with caution and under the guidance of a qualified herbalist or healthcare provider, especially if you are taking medications or have underlying health conditions. Always seek professional advice before using echinacea as a natural remedy.

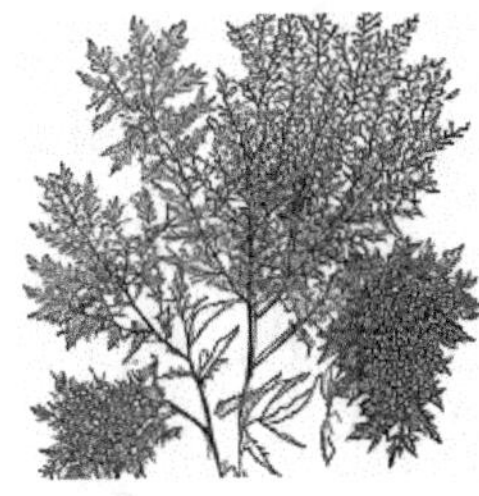 **Elderberry (Sambucus)** is the fruit of the elder tree or shrub. These dark purple to black berries have a long history of medicinal and culinary use. Here is an overview of elderberry, including its historical use, medicinal uses, visual identification, growth conditions, reparation, and potential health benefits.

Historical Use: Elderberries have been used for centuries in traditional medicine systems, particularly in Europe and North America. In the past, various parts of the elder tree, including berries, leaves, flowers, and bark, have been used for their potential health benefits.

Medicinal Uses: Elderberries are valued for their potential health benefits and are known for their various uses in traditional medicine. Immune Support: Elderberries are rich in antioxidants, vitamins, and flavonoids, which are believed to support the immune system and help the body defend against illnesses, particularly colds and flu. Respiratory Health: Elderberry is traditionally used to alleviate symptoms of respiratory infections and conditions, such as coughs and congestion. Antiviral Properties: Some studies suggest that compounds in elderberries may have antiviral effects and can inhibit the replication of certain viruses. Anti-Inflammatory Effects: Elderberry may help reduce inflammation and promote overall well-being. Digestive Health: Elderberries have been used for digestive complaints, such as constipation and indigestion.

Visual Identification: Elderberries are small, round, and typically dark purple to black when ripe. They grow in clusters on the elder tree (Sambucus), a deciduous shrub or small tree. The elderberry shrub or tree features pinnately compound leaves and produce small white or cream-colored flowers in the spring, followed by the formation of the berries in late summer to early Autumn.

Growth Conditions: Elderberries are easy to grow and can be cultivated in various regions with the right conditions. Here are some factors to consider when growing elderberries: Geographical Area: Elderberries are found in various parts of the world and are well-suited to temperate climates. Cultivation: Elderberries are grown from cuttings or young plants and require well-drained soil and proper spacing. Climate: They grow best in areas with a distinct winter, as they require a period of winter dormancy. Soil: Elderberries prefer fertile, loamy soil with good drainage.

Preparation and Health Benefits: Elderberries can be consumed in various forms to enjoy their potential health benefits. Elderberry Syrup: Elderberry syrup is a common preparation that can be taken as a natural remedy for immune support during the cold and flu season. It is available commercially, or you can make your own using dried Elderberries. Elderberry Tea: Dried elderberries can be used to prepare elderberry tea, which is enjoyed for its potential immune-boosting properties. Elderberry Extract: Liquid elderberry extracts or tinctures are available and can be used as directed by a healthcare provider or herbalist. Elderberry Jam or Jelly: Elderberries are sometimes used to make jams, jellies, or pies for a delicious way to enjoy their flavor and potential health benefits. Supplements: Elderberry supplements, such as capsules or gummies, are available in many health stores and can be used according to the manufacturer's instructions.

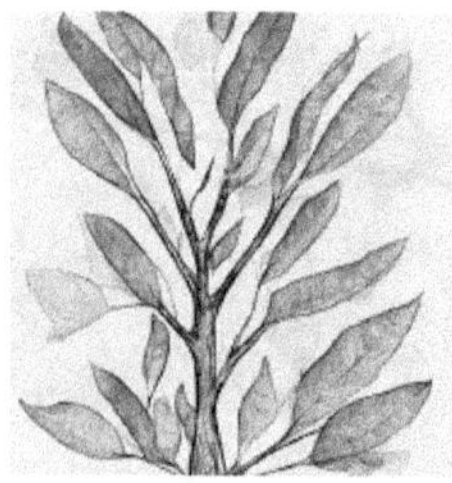

Eucalyptus (Eucalyptus globulus) is a versatile and aromatic tree native to Australia and Tasmania. It is known for its medicinal properties, primarily concerning respiratory health, and is used in various products such as essential oils, cough drops, and chest rubs. Here is a detailed overview of eucalyptus, including its historical use, medicinal properties, visual identification, growth conditions, care, precautions, and potential health benefits.

Historical Use: medicinal properties, particularly in addressing respiratory ailments. It was introduced to other parts of the world in the 18th century.

Medicinal Properties: Eucalyptus is traditionally used for its potential health benefits, including Respiratory Health. It is well-known for relieving symptoms of respiratory conditions, such as coughs, colds, and congestion.

Anti-Inflammatory: Eucalyptus has anti-inflammatory properties that can help reduce inflammation and pain. Antibacterial: It may have antibacterial properties and can be used topically on wounds. Aromatherapy: Eucalyptus essential oil is widely used in aromatherapy for its refreshing and invigorating scent.

Visual Identification: Eucalyptus trees can be recognized by the following characteristics: Tall, evergreen trees with lance-shaped leaves. White, cream, or pinkish flowers. Distinctive, woody fruits are often referred to as "gum nuts."

Growth Conditions: Eucalyptus trees are native to Australia and thrive in sunny, dry climates with well-drained soil. They are adapted to withstand drought and are known for their rapid growth.

Care: Eucalyptus trees can be grown from seeds or cuttings. They require full sun and well-drained soil. Pruning may be necessary to control growth and encourage bushier growth.

Precautions: Eucalyptus essential oil is safe for external use when diluted but should not be ingested. Ingesting eucalyptus oil can be toxic and potentially fatal, so it should be used with caution and only under the guidance of a healthcare provider. Eucalyptus oil should not be applied to the face or chest of young children, particularly infants, as it can lead to respiratory distress. Consult a healthcare provider before using eucalyptus for specific health concerns, especially if you have underlying health conditions.

Eucalyptus is a valuable herb for respiratory health and has a variety of applications, primarily in the form of essential oil and topical products. It should be used cautiously, and eucalyptus essential oil should always be appropriately diluted when applied to the skin. Consult with a healthcare provider before using eucalyptus for specific health concerns, especially if you have underlying health conditions or are using it with children.

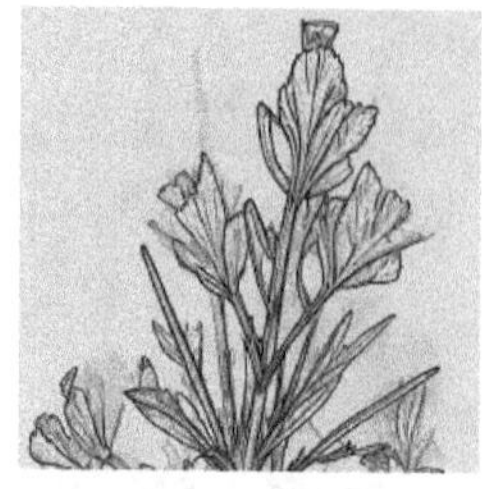

Evening primrose oil (Oenothera biennis) is derived from the evening primrose plant's seeds, a wildflower native to North America. The oil is known for its potential medicinal benefits, particularly for women's health, skin health, and reducing inflammation. Here is a detailed overview of evening primrose oil, including its historical use, medicinal properties, visual identification, growth conditions, care, precautions, and potential health benefits.

Historical Use: Evening primrose has a history of use among Indigenous North American tribes for its potential medicinal properties. It gained popularity in the 20th century as a dietary supplement and natural remedy.

Medicinal Properties: Evening primrose oil is traditionally used for potential health benefits, including women's health. It is often used to alleviate symptoms of premenstrual syndrome (PMS) symptoms and menopause, such as breast tenderness and hot flashes. Skin Health: Evening primrose oil supports skin health and may help alleviate conditions like eczema and acne. Anti-Inflammatory: It may have anti-inflammatory properties that can help reduce inflammation and pain. Rheumatoid Arthritis: Some studies have suggested that evening primrose oil may benefit individuals with rheumatoid arthritis.

Visual Identification: Evening primrose plants can be recognized by the following characteristics: tall, slender plants with lance-shaped leaves. Bright yellow, four-petaled flowers that bloom in the evening. Tubular seed pods containing oil-rich seeds.

Growth Conditions: Evening primrose is native to North America and thrives in well-drained soil and full sun. It is often found in fields, meadows, and along roadsides. Care: Evening primrose can be grown from seeds or seedlings. It requires full sun and well-drained soil. Adequate watering and soil preparation are important for successful cultivation.

Precautions: Evening primrose oil is considered safe when used as directed, but it should not be ingested in excessive amounts. Some individuals may experience mild gastrointestinal discomfort or allergic reactions. Evening primrose oil may interact with certain medications, particularly blood-thinning drugs, and should be used with caution by individuals taking such medications. Consult with a healthcare provider before using evening primrose oil for specific health concerns, especially if you have underlying health conditions or are taking medications. Evening primrose oil is a popular dietary supplement and natural remedy, particularly for women's health and skin conditions. It should be used with caution and under the guidance of a qualified healthcare provider, especially if you are taking medications or have underlying health conditions. Always seek professional advice before using evening primrose oil as a natural remedy.

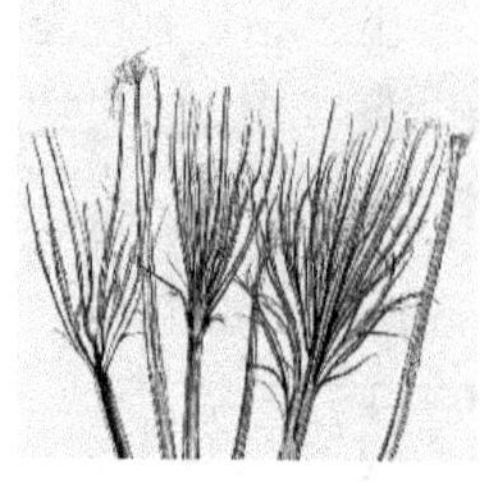

Fennel (Foeniculum vulgare)

is a flowering plant with feathery leaves and aromatic seeds. It is native to the Mediterranean region but is now cultivated and grown worldwide. Fennel is used for its culinary and medicinal properties and has been appreciated for its potential health benefits for centuries. Here is a detailed overview of fennel, including its historical use, culinary uses, medicinal properties, visual identification, growth conditions, care, precautions, and potential health benefits:

Historical Use: Fennel has a long history of use in various cultures for culinary and medicinal purposes. It was used by ancient Greeks and Romans for its aromatic qualities and believed to have medicinal properties.

Culinary Uses: Fennel is used in various culinary applications, including Cooking. The bulb, stalks, leaves, and fennel seeds are used in various dishes, from salads to soups and stews. Flavoring: Fennel seeds are used as a spice in many cuisines, imparting a sweet, licorice-like flavor to foods. Herbal Teas: Fennel seeds are used to prepare herbal teas, often used for digestive purposes.

Medicinal Properties: Fennel is traditionally used for its potential health benefits, including Digestive Health: It is believed to help with indigestion, bloating, and gas. Anti-Inflammatory: Fennel has anti-inflammatory properties and may help reduce inflammation.
Respiratory Health: It alleviates respiratory issues like coughs and bronchitis. Menstrual Health: Fennel tea is often used to alleviate menstrual discomfort and cramps.

Visual Identification: Fennel plants can be recognized by the following characteristics: Tall, feathery green leaves. Yellow flowers that grow in umbrella-like clusters. A bulbous, white, or pale green base that resembles celery but has distinct licorice flavor.

Growth Conditions: Fennel can be grown in various regions and climates. It prefers well-drained soil, full sun, and moderate moisture.

Care: Fennel can be grown from seeds and requires well-prepared soil. Adequate spacing and thinning are essential to promote proper bulb development. Regular watering is necessary to prevent bolting (premature flowering).

Precautions: Fennel is considered safe for most people when consumed in moderation. However, some individuals may be sensitive to it and experience allergic reactions. Fennel may interact with certain medications, particularly blood-thinning drugs, and should be used with caution by individuals taking such medications. Consult with a healthcare provider before using fennel for specific health concerns, especially if you have underlying health conditions or are taking medications. Fennel is a versatile herb and vegetable with many culinary and potential health benefits. It is especially known for its digestive and respiratory health benefits. It should be used cautiously, and fennel tea is often used for its medicinal properties. Consult a healthcare provider before using fennel for specific health concerns, especially if you have allergies or underlying health conditions.

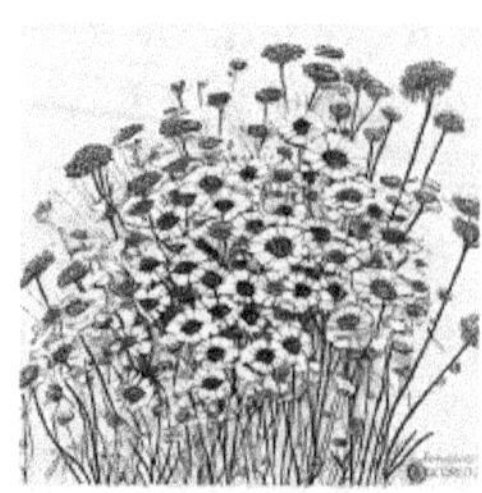

Feverfew (Tanacetum parthenium)

is an herb known for its historical use in traditional medicine and potential health benefits. Here is an overview of feverfew, including its historical use, medicinal uses, visual identification, growth conditions, preparation, and potential health benefits.

Historical Use: Feverfew has a long history of use in traditional medicine, particularly European folk medicine. It was traditionally used for various health purposes, including managing fever, migraines, and inflammatory conditions. The name "feverfew" is derived from its historical use to reduce fevers.

Medicinal Uses: Feverfew is valued for its potential medicinal properties and has been used for various health benefits. Migraine Management: Feverfew has been traditionally used to help prevent and alleviate migraine headaches. Some research suggests that it may reduce the frequency and severity of migraines. Anti-Inflammatory Effects: Feverfew is believed to have anti-inflammatory properties, which may be beneficial for various inflammatory conditions. Arthritis Support: It has been used to alleviate symptoms of arthritis and other musculoskeletal conditions. Fever Reduction: As the name implies, feverfew has historically been used to reduce fever, although it is less commonly used today.

Visual Identification: Feverfew is a perennial herb with distinctive characteristics. Leaves: When crushed, the leaves are deeply lobed and have a pungent, slightly bitter aroma. Flowers: Feverfew produces small, daisy-like flowers with white petals and a yellow center. The flowers are typically found in clusters. Height: The plant can grow up to 2-3 feet tall. Growth Conditions: Feverfew can be cultivated in various regions with the right conditions. Geographical Area: It is native to the Balkans and throughout Europe. It can be cultivated in other temperate regions as well. Cultivation: Feverfew is typically grown from seeds, cuttings, or young plants and thrives in well-drained soil with good air circulation. Climate: It prefers temperate climates with moderate rainfall. Soil: Well-draining soil with a slightly alkaline to neutral pH is ideal.

Preparation and Health Benefits: Feverfew can be consumed or used in various forms to enjoy its potential health benefits. Feverfew Supplements: Feverfew is available in supplement form, including capsules and tablets. The recommended dosage varies, so it is important to follow the product label instructions or consult a healthcare provider.

Feverfew Tea: Dried feverfew leaves can be used to make feverfew tea. This herbal tea is sometimes consumed for its potential benefits, such as migraine relief. To prepare the tea, steep one teaspoon of dried feverfew leaves in a cup of hot water for about 10-15 minutes, then strain and drink.

Tinctures: Feverfew tinctures are liquid extracts and can be used as directed by a healthcare provider. It is crucial to use feverfew responsibly and consult with a healthcare provider, especially if you are pregnant, nursing, or taking medications.

The use of feverfew for migraine prevention should be discussed with a healthcare provider, as individual responses may vary. Obtaining feverfew products from reputable sources ensures quality and safety.

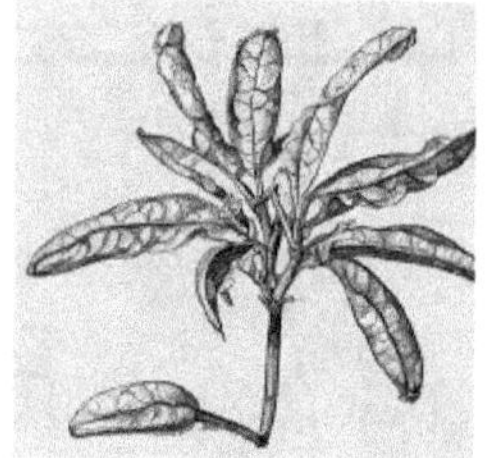

Garcinia cambogia (Garcinia gummi-gutta), also known as Malabar tamarind, is a tropical fruit native to Southeast Asia. It has recently gained popularity as a potential dietary supplement for weight management. Here is a detailed overview of Garcinia cambogia, including its historical use, medicinal properties, visual identification, growth conditions, care, precautions, and potential health benefits.

Historical Use: Garcinia cambogia has a long history of use in traditional Southeast Asian cuisine, particularly in curries and other dishes. It has also been used in Ayurvedic medicine for digestive support.

Medicinal Properties: Garcinia cambogia is primarily promoted for its potential health benefits, including weight management. It is often marketed as a dietary supplement for weight loss, with some studies suggesting it may help reduce body weight and appetite. Appetite Suppression: Some of the active compounds in Garcinia cambogia are believed to have an appetite-suppressing effect. Cholesterol and Blood Sugar Support: There is some evidence that Garcinia cambogia may help improve cholesterol and blood sugar levels.

Visual Identification: Garcinia cambogia fruit and tree can be recognized by the following characteristics: It is a small, pumpkin-shaped fruit with a yellow or greenish rind. Inside the fruit, there are typically several seeds surrounded by a fleshy, sour pulp. The tree itself has evergreen leaves and a dense canopy.

Growth Conditions: Garcinia cambogia is tropical and requires warm, humid conditions to thrive. It is typically grown in regions with a tropical or subtropical climate.

Care: Garcinia cambogia can be grown from seeds or cuttings, but it requires specific tropical conditions to grow successfully. Adequate sunlight, warmth, and well-drained, fertile soil are essential for its Cultivation.

Precautions: While Garcinia cambogia is considered safe for short-term use, it should not be consumed excessively. Some individuals may experience mild side effects, including digestive discomfort or headaches. Garcinia cambogia supplements should be used cautiously, as their safety and effectiveness vary. Consult with a healthcare provider before using them, especially if you have underlying health conditions or are taking medications.

Garcinia cambogia has gained attention primarily as a dietary supplement for weight management. It should be used cautiously, and choosing high-quality supplements is essential if you try them. Always consult a healthcare provider before using Garcinia cambogia for specific health concerns, especially if you have underlying health conditions or are taking medications.

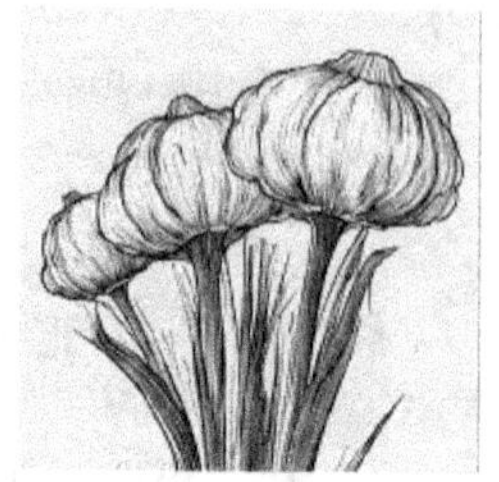

Garlic (Allium sativum) is a popular and widely used herb with a long history of culinary and medicinal use. It is well-known for its distinctive flavor and aroma, as well as its potential health benefits. Here is a detailed overview of garlic, including its historical use, culinary uses, medicinal properties, visual identification, growth conditions, care, precautions, and potential health benefits.

Historical Use: Garlic has been used for thousands of years in various cultures for culinary and medicinal purposes. It was used by the ancient Egyptians, Greeks, and Romans and has been highly regarded for its potential health benefits.

Culinary Uses: Garlic is a versatile ingredient used in various culinary applications, including Flavoring. It adds a distinctive, savory flavor to various dishes, from soups and sauces to roasted meats and vegetables. Spice: Garlic can be used as a spice in multiple forms, including minced, crushed, or in the form of garlic powder. Condiments: Garlic is used to make condiments such as garlic butter, aioli, and garlic-infused oils. Pickling: Garlic cloves can be pickled and added to recipes or used as a condiment.

Medicinal Properties: Garlic is traditionally used for its potential health benefits, including Cardiovascular Health. It may help lower blood pressure and reduce the risk of heart disease. Antibacterial and Antifungal: Garlic has natural antimicrobial properties and may help combat infections. Anti-Inflammatory: It is believed to have anti-inflammatory properties. Immune Support: Garlic may help support the immune system and reduce the severity and duration of colds and flu.

Visual Identification: Garlic plants can be recognized by the following characteristics: Bulbous underground root structure composed of individual cloves. Long, slender leaves that grow in a rosette from the central bulb. Flowering stalk with small, white, or pink flowers.

Growth Conditions: Garlic is typically grown in regions with cold winters and warm summers. It requires well-drained soil and full sun.

Care: Garlic is commonly propagated by planting individual cloves. Adequate spacing and mulching are essential for successful growth. Regular watering and proper maintenance are necessary to prevent diseases and ensure bulb development.

Precautions: Garlic is safe for most people when consumed in moderation as food. Some individuals may experience digestive discomfort or allergic reactions. Garlic supplements or concentrated forms should be used with caution, especially by individuals taking blood-thinning medications or undergoing surgery. Consult with a healthcare provider before using garlic supplements for specific health concerns, especially if you have underlying health conditions or are taking medications.

Garlic is a beloved culinary ingredient and is appreciated for its potential health benefits, particularly in relation to cardiovascular health and immune support. It is safe to use as a food but should be used with caution in supplement form.

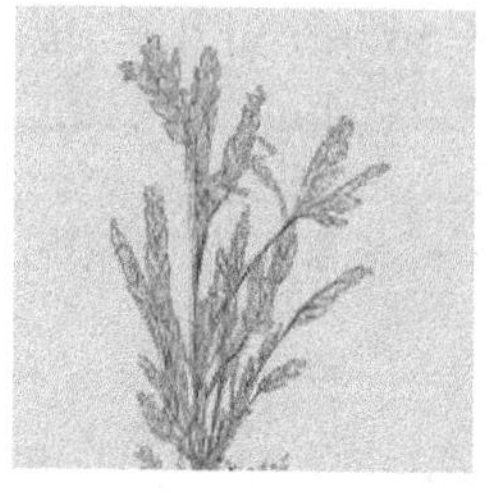

Ginger (Zingiber officinale) is a well-known and widely used spice and medicinal herb with a long history of use in various cultures worldwide. It is renowned for its distinct flavor, aroma, and potential health benefits. Here is a detailed overview of ginger, including its historical use, culinary uses, medicinal properties, visual identification, growth conditions, care, precautions, and potential health benefits.

Historical Use: Ginger has been used for centuries in traditional medicine systems, particularly in Ayurveda and Traditional Chinese Medicine. It was also highly valued as a spice and trade commodity.

Culinary Uses: Ginger is a versatile ingredient used in various culinary applications, including flavoring. It adds a spicy, pungent flavor to dishes, such as curries, stir-fries, and baked goods.
teas: Ginger can be used to prepare ginger tea or chai, which is enjoyed for its warming and soothing qualities. Candied Ginger: Ginger can be candied or crystallized and used as a sweet snack or dessert. Pickled Ginger: Thinly sliced ginger is pickled and served as a condiment with sushi.

Medicinal Properties: Ginger is traditionally used for its potential health benefits, including Digestive Health: It is well-known for its ability to alleviate nausea, including motion sickness, morning sickness, and nausea caused by chemotherapy. Anti-Inflammatory: Ginger has anti-inflammatory properties that may help reduce inflammation and pain. Arthritis Relief: Some individuals use ginger to alleviate symptoms of osteoarthritis and rheumatoid arthritis. Respiratory Health: Ginger may help relieve symptoms of respiratory conditions like colds and bronchitis.

Visual Identification: Ginger plants can be recognized by the following characteristics: Tall, reed-like stems with lance-shaped leaves. Cone-like inflorescences with yellow or white flowers. Underground rhizomes (roots) that are harvested for use.

Growth Conditions: Ginger is a tropical plant and requires warm, humid conditions to thrive. It is typically grown in regions with a tropical or subtropical climate.

Care: Ginger can be grown from rhizomes or seeds. Adequate sunlight, warmth, and well-drained, fertile soil are essential for its cultivation. Regular watering and proper care are necessary to ensure successful growth.

Precautions: Ginger is considered safe when consumed as food or as a spice in culinary dishes. Some individuals may experience mild side effects, such as heartburn or digestive discomfort. Ginger supplements should be used cautiously, especially by individuals taking blood-thinning medications or undergoing surgery. Consult with a healthcare provider before using ginger supplements for specific health concerns, especially if you have underlying health conditions or are taking medications.

Ginger is a beloved spice and natural remedy, well-regarded for its culinary versatility and potential health benefits, particularly in relation to digestive health and reducing inflammation. It is safe to use as a food but should be used cautiously in supplement form. Consult with a healthcare provider before using ginger supplements for specific health concerns, especially if you have underlying health conditions or are taking medications.

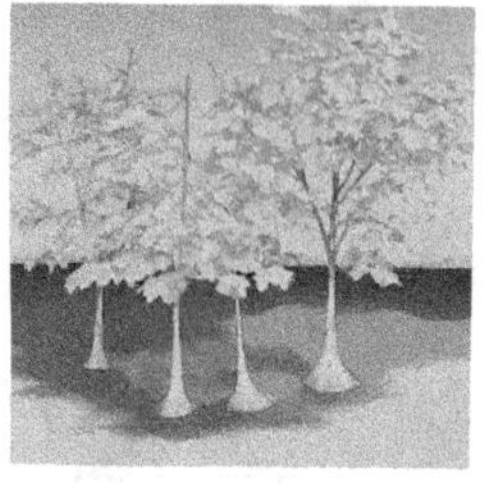

Ginkgo biloba, commonly known as ginkgo or maidenhair tree, is a unique and ancient tree species with a long history of traditional use in various cultures. It is known for its distinctive fan-shaped leaves and is valued for its potential medicinal properties. Here is a detailed overview of ginkgo biloba, including its historical use, visual identification, medicinal properties, precautions, and potential health benefits.

Historical Use: Ginkgo biloba is one of the oldest tree species on Earth, dating back over 200 million years. Traditional use of ginkgo can be traced to China, where it has been used in traditional Chinese medicine for centuries. It has been historically used to improve memory cognition and to address various health issues.

Visual Identification: Ginkgo biloba is a large, deciduous tree. It has distinctive fan-shaped leaves with a unique bilobed structure. The leaves turn a bright golden yellow in the fall. The tree produces small, plum-like seeds.

Medicinal Properties: Ginkgo biloba is primarily known for its potential cognitive and circulatory benefits, including Improving Cognitive Function. Some studies suggest it may help enhance memory, concentration, and cognitive function, especially in older adults. Circulatory Support: Ginkgo may promote healthy blood circulation and support cardiovascular health. Antioxidant Properties: It contains antioxidants that help protect cells from oxidative stress.

Precautions: While considered safe, ginkgo biloba may interact with certain medications, particularly blood thinners. Some individuals may experience side effects such as digestive upset or headaches. It should be used under the guidance of a healthcare provider, especially if you have underlying health conditions or are taking medications.

Ginkgo biloba is commonly available in the form of supplements, extracts, and herbal remedies. It is often recommended to support cognitive health and circulation. Consult with a healthcare provider before using ginkgo biloba supplements, especially if you have underlying health conditions or are taking medications.

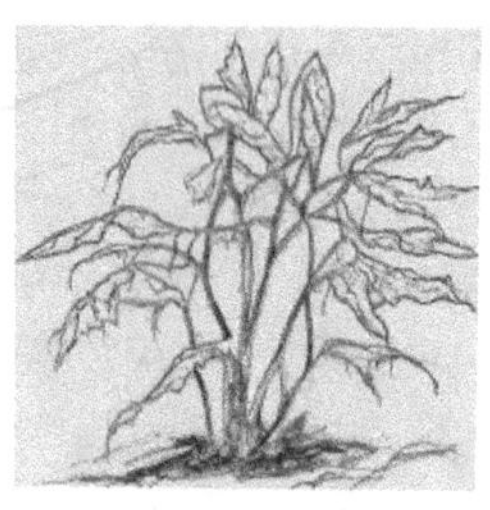

Ginseng (Panax quinquefolius)

is a perennial herb native to North America and is highly regarded for its potential medicinal properties. It is one of the several ginseng species known for its adaptogenic qualities and use in traditional medicine. Here is a detailed overview of American ginseng, including its historical use, medicinal properties, visual identification, growth conditions, care, precautions, and potential health benefits.

Historical Use: American ginseng has a long history of use among Native American tribes and in traditional herbal medicine. It was valued for its potential health benefits and adaptogenic properties, helping the body adapt to stress.

Medicinal Properties: American ginseng is traditionally used for its potential health benefits, including adaptogenic: It is onsidered an adaptogen, which means it may help the body adapt to stress and improve resilience. Energy and Stamina: Ginseng is often used to increase energy levels, enhance stamina, and combat fatigue. Cognitive Function: Some studies suggest that ginseng may support cognitive function, including memory and mental alertness. Immune Support: It may help strengthen the immune system and reduce the risk of infections.

Visual Identification: American ginseng plants can be recognized by the following characteristics: Compound leaves with five leaflets. Greenish-white, umbrella-like clusters of flowers. Small, red berries.

Growth Conditions: American ginseng gro
woodlands with well-drained, loamy soil. It is rich, moist
the eastern United States, particularly in the Appa. found in
region.

Care: American ginseng is typically propagated by plan
Growing successfully requires specific conditions, eeds.
shade, moisture, and soil acidity. Ginseng is a slow-growing
and may take several years to mature.

Precautions: American ginseng is considered safe when used as directed but should not be consumed excessively. Some individuals may experience side effects, including digestive discomfort or insomnia. American ginseng may interact with certain medications, particularly anticoagulants, and should be used cautiously by individuals taking such medications. Consult with a healthcare provider before using American ginseng for specific health concerns, especially if you have underlying health conditions or are taking medications. American ginseng is a valued herb known for its adaptogenic qualities and potential health benefits, particularly concerning energy, cognitive function, and immune support. It should be used cautiously and under the guidance of a qualified herbalist or healthcare provider, especially if you are taking medications or have underlying health conditions. Always seek professional advice before using American ginseng as a natural remedy.

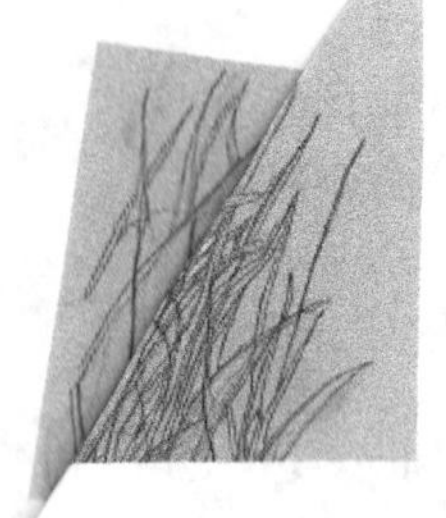

Goldenseal (Hydrastis canadensis) is a perennial herb native to North America and known for its potential medicinal properties, particularly in traditional Native American medicine. It has a long history of use and is highly regarded for its potential health benefits.

Historical Use: Goldenseal has a rich history of use among Native American tribes, particularly the Cherokee, who used it for medicinal purposes. It was introduced to European settlers in the 18th century and gained popularity in Western herbal medicine.

Medicinal Properties: Goldenseal is traditionally used for its potential health benefits, including Antibacterial: It is believed to have natural antibacterial properties and was historically used to address infections. Anti-Inflammatory: Goldenseal may have anti-inflammatory properties that can help reduce inflammation and pain. Immune Support: It supports the immune system and general health. Digestive Health: Goldenseal is believed to help with digestive issues like diarrhea and indigestion.

Visual Identification: Goldenseal plants can be recognized by the following characteristics: Low-growing herb with palmately lobed leaves. Single, nodding, white flower with green sepals. Bright red, knotty rhizomes (roots) are typically used in herbal preparations.

Growth Conditions: Goldenseal grows in rich, moist woodlands with well-drained, loamy soil. It is typically found in the eastern United States, particularly in the Appalachian region.

Care: Goldenseal is typically propagated by planting rhizomes. To grow successfully requires specific conditions, including shade, moisture, and soil acidity. Goldenseal is slow-growing and may take several years to mature.

Precautions: Goldenseal is considered safe when used as directed but should not be consumed excessively. Some individuals may experience side effects, including digestive discomfort or allergic reactions. It may interact with certain medications, particularly blood-thinning drugs, and should be used cautiously by individuals taking such medications. Consult with a healthcare provider before using goldenseal for specific health concerns, especially if you have underlying health conditions or are taking medications.

Goldenseal is a valued herb known for its potential antibacterial and anti-inflammatory properties, among other health benefits. It should be used with caution and under the guidance of a qualified herbalist or healthcare provider, especially if you are taking medications or have underlying health conditions. Always seek professional advice before using goldenseal as a natural remedy.

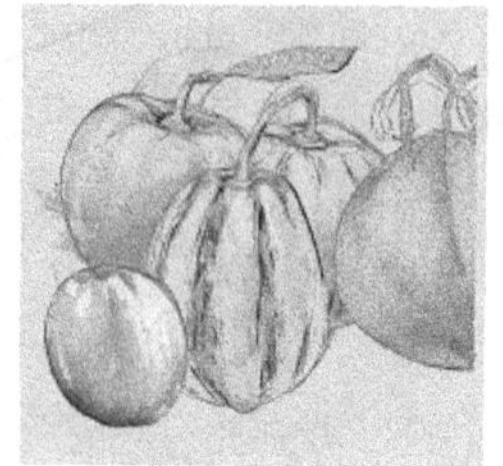

Grapefruit seed extract (GSE) is a supplement derived from grapefruit seeds, pulp, and white membranes (Citrus paradisi). It is known for its potential medicinal properties and is often used as a natural remedy. Here is a detailed overview of grapefruit seed extract, including its historical use, medicinal properties, visual identification, growth conditions, care, precautions, and potential health benefits.

Historical Use: Grapefruit seed extract gained popularity in the 1980s as a dietary Supplement and natural remedy, particularly for its potential antimicrobial properties.

Medicinal Properties: Grapefruit seed extract is traditionally used for its potential health benefits, Including Antimicrobial: It is believed to have natural antimicrobial properties and is often used for its ability to combat bacterial and fungal infections. Antioxidant: GSE contains antioxidants, which may help reduce oxidative stress and inflammation. Immune Support: It supports the immune system and overall health. Digestive Health: Some individuals use GSE to alleviate digestive issues like diarrhea and irritable bowel syndrome.

Visual Identification: Grapefruit seed extract is not derived directly from the fruit but from the seeds and pulp, which are typically small, hard, and pale.

Growth Conditions: Grapefruits are grown in subtropical and tropical regions worldwide. They require a warm climate, well-drained soil, and adequate sunlight for proper growth.

Care: Grapefruit trees need specific conditions, such as warmth and protection from frost. Proper pruning and pest control are essential for successful cultivation. Regular watering and soil management are necessary for healthy tree growth.

Precautions:
Grapefruit seed extract is considered safe when used as directed but should not be consumed excessively. Some individuals may experience side effects, including gastrointestinal discomfort or allergic reactions. Grapefruit seed extract may interact with certain medications, particularly blood-thinning drugs and medications affected by the CYP450 enzyme system. It can increase the concentration of some drugs in the bloodstream.

Consult with a healthcare provider before using grapefruit seed extract for specific health concerns, especially if you have underlying health conditions or are taking medications.

Grapefruit seed extract is a dietary supplement and natural remedy with potential antimicrobial and antioxidant properties. It should be used cautiously, and it is essential to consult with a healthcare provider before using it, especially if you are taking medications or have underlying health conditions. Always seek professional advice before using grapefruit seed extract as a natural remedy.

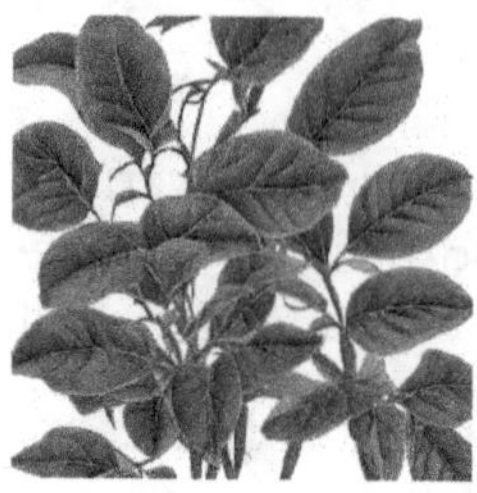

Green tea derived from the leaves of the Camellia sinensis plant leaves is a popular beverage enjoyed worldwide and known for its potential health benefits. Here is a detailed overview of green tea, including its historical use, preparation, medicinal properties, visual identification, growth conditions, care, precautions, and potential health benefits.

Historical Use: Green tea has a long history of use, dating back over 4,000 years in China, where it originated. It has been valued for its taste, aroma, and potential health benefits.

Preparation: To prepare green tea, follow these general steps: Boil Water: Heat fresh, cold water to just below boiling, around 175°F to 185°F (80°C to 85°C). Choose Tea: Select good-quality green tea leaves or tea bags. Infusion: Place the tea leaves or tea bag in a teapot or cup. Pour the hot water over the tea. Steeping: Allow the tea to steep for 1-3 minutes, depending on your preference for strength. Serve: Remove the tea leaves or tea bag and enjoy.

Medicinal Properties: Green tea is traditionally used for its potential health benefits, including Antioxidant Properties: Green tea is rich in antioxidants called catechins, which may help protect cells from damage caused by free radicals.

Heart Health: Some studies suggest that green tea may help lower the risk of heart disease by reducing harmful cholesterol levels and improving blood vessel function. Weight Management: Green tea is believed to support weight management by increasing metabolism and fat oxidation.

Cognitive Function: It may support cognitive function and memory.

Oral Health: Green tea has natural antibacterial properties and may help improve oral health.

Visual Identification: Camellia sinensis plants can be recognized by the following characteristics: Glossy, dark green leaves with serrated edges—small, white, fragrant flowers with yellow centers. Tea plants are typically pruned and maintained as shrubs.

Growth Conditions: Camellia sinensis prefers specific conditions for optimal growth: Subtropical or tropical climate. Well-drained, slightly acidic soil. Full or partial sun exposure.

Care: Proper pruning and maintenance are essential for tea plant cultivation. Protection from frost or extreme temperatures is necessary for healthy growth. Adequate moisture and soil management are crucial for the tea plant's well-being.

Precautions: Green tea is considered safe when consumed in moderation. Excessive consumption may lead to caffeine-related side effects, such as insomnia or jitters. Some individuals may experience gastrointestinal discomfort. Green tea supplements should be used with caution, especially by individuals sensitive to caffeine. Consult with a healthcare provider for specific health concerns, especially if you have underlying health conditions or are taking medications.

Green tea is a widely consumed and beloved beverage known for its potential health benefits, particularly in relation to its antioxidant properties and potential to support heart health and weight management. It is safe when consumed in moderation but should be used cautiously in supplement form. Consult with a healthcare provider before using green tea supplements for specific health concerns, especially if you have underlying health conditions or are taking medications.

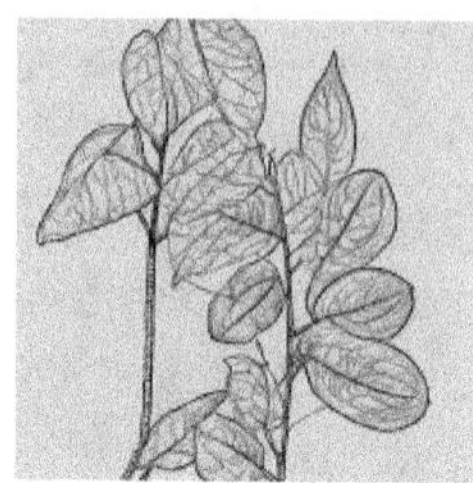

Gymnema (Gymnema sylvestre) is a plant native to the tropical forests of India and Africa and is known for its potential medicinal properties, particularly in traditional Ayurvedic medicine. It has been used for centuries for its potential health benefits. Here is a detailed overview of Gymnema, including its historical use, medicinal properties, visual identification, growth conditions, care, precautions, and potential health benefits:

Historical Use: Gymnema has a long history of use in Ayurvedic medicine, where it is known as "Gurmar" or "sugar destroyer." It was traditionally used to support blood sugar balance.

Medicinal Properties: Gymnema is traditionally used for potential health benefits, including Blood Sugar Control. Gymnema is believed to help lower blood sugar levels by reducing the absorption of sugar in the intestines and increasing glucose uptake by cells. Appetite Suppression: It may help reduce cravings for sweet foods, which can benefit weight management.
Digestive Health: Some individuals use Gymnema to support digestive health and alleviate symptoms like indigestion and constipation. Anti-Inflammatory: It is believed to have anti-inflammatory properties that can help reduce inflammation and pain.

Visual Identification: Gymnema plants can be recognized by the following characteristics: Climbing or spreading woody vines with small, oblong leaves. Clusters of small, yellow flowers. Seed pods that contain oval-shaped seeds.

338

Growth Conditions: Gymnema is a tropical plant and requires warm, humid conditions to thrive. It is typically found in regions with a tropical or subtropical climate.

Care: Gymnema can be grown from seeds or cuttings. Adequate sunlight, warmth, and well-drained, fertile soil are essential for its cultivation. Regular watering and proper care are necessary for successful growth.

Precautions: Gymnema is considered safe when used as directed. It is not a substitute for prescribed diabetes medications, and a healthcare provider should monitor its use should be monitored by a healthcare provider. Some individuals may experience side effects, including digestive discomfort.

Consult with a healthcare provider before using Gymnema for specific health concerns, especially if you have diabetes or are taking medications. Gymnema is an herb with potential blood sugar-regulating properties, and it is traditionally used to support blood sugar balance and reduce sugar cravings. It should be used cautiously, and it is essential to consult with a healthcare provider, particularly if you have diabetes or are taking medications. Always seek professional advice before using Gymnema as a natural remedy.

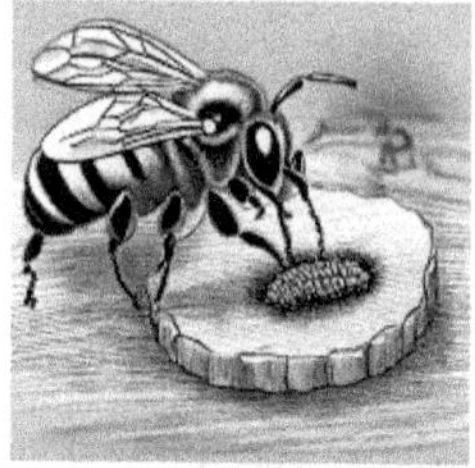

Honey is a natural sweet substance produced by bees from the nectar of flowers. It has been used for thousands of years by humans as both a sweetener and a traditional remedy. Honey is valued for its unique taste, aroma, and potential health benefits. Here is a detailed overview of honey, including its historical use, culinary uses, medicinal properties, visual identification, production, precautions, and potential health benefits.

Historical Use: Honey has a rich history of use that dates back thousands of years. It was used by ancient civilizations, including the Egyptians, Greeks, and Romans, as a sweetener and a natural remedy for various ailments.

Culinary Uses: Honey is used in a wide range of culinary applications, including sweetener: It is used as a natural sweetener in beverages, baking, and cooking. Condiment: Honey can be drizzled on yogurt, fruits, or desserts. Preservative: Its natural composition, including low water content and acidity, makes it a preservative for fruits, vegetables, and other foods.

Medicinal Properties: Honey is traditionally used for its potential health benefits, including Cough and Sore Throat. Honey can help soothe coughs and sore throats, making it a common ingredient in many over-the-counter cough syrups. Wound Healing: It has natural antimicrobial properties and has been used topically to aid wound healing. Antioxidant: Honey contains antioxidants that help protect cells from damage caused by free radicals.

Digestive Health: Some individuals use honey to alleviate digestive issues like constipation.

Visual Identification: Honey is a thick, sticky, golden to amber-colored liquid with a distinctive sweet aroma. Its appearance can vary depending on the type of nectar and flowers bees use.

Production: Honey is produced by honeybees, who collect nectar from flowers and store it in their hives. The bees process the nectar and transform it into honey by adding enzymes and reducing the water content. Once the honey is sufficiently concentrated, the bees seal it in honeycomb cells.

Precautions: Honey is considered safe when consumed by most people, but it should not be given to infants under one year of age due to the risk of botulism. Some individuals may experience allergic reactions to honey. It is essential to use raw honey cautiously in individuals with pollen allergies, as it may contain traces of pollen. Consult with a healthcare provider before using honey as a natural remedy for specific
health concerns.

Honey is a beloved natural sweetener with potential health benefits, particularly for soothing coughs and sore throats. It is safe and can be a healthier alternative to refined sugar. However, it should be used with caution in certain situations and under the guidance of a healthcare provider, especially in infants and individuals with pollen allergies.

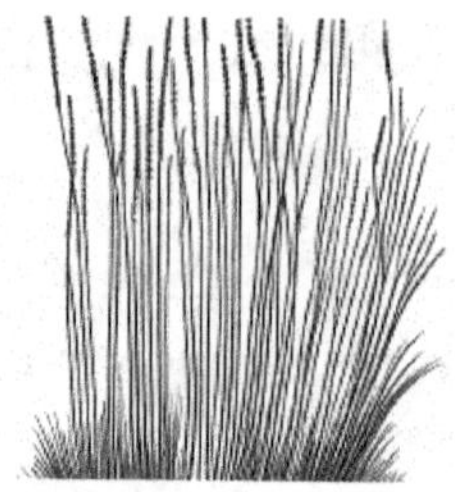

Horsetail (Equisetum arvense) is a perennial plant used for centuries in traditional medicine for its potential health benefits. It is known for its unique appearance and is often used to make herbal infusions. Here is a detailed overview of horsetail, including its historical use, medicinal properties, visual identification, growth conditions, care, precautions, and potential health benefits.

Historical Use: Horsetail has a long history of use in traditional herbal medicine, particularly in Europe and Asia. It was used for various purposes, including promoting hair and nail growth, wound healing, and as a diuretic.

Medicinal Properties: Horsetail is traditionally used for its potential health benefits, including diuretics. It may increase urine output and reduce water retention. Skin and Hair Health: Horsetail is believed to support skin and hair health due to its high silica content. Wound Healing: It has been used topically to help wounds heal. Anti-Inflammatory: Some individuals use horsetail to alleviate inflammation and pain.

Visual Identification: Horsetail plants can be recognized by the following characteristics: Hollow, segmented stems with a jointed appearance resembling a horse's tail. Delicate, needle-like leaves.
Cone-like structures at the top of the stems which contain spores.
Growth Conditions: Horsetail typically grows in moist, well-drained soil in various regions, including North America, Europe, and Asia. It can be found in wetlands, meadows, and along   stream   banks.

Care: Horsetail is a hardy, low-maintenance plant and can be invasive if not controlled. Adequate moisture and soil management are necessary for healthy growth. Proper pruning and maintenance can help prevent overgrowth.

Precautions: Horsetail is considered safe when used as directed but should not be consumed excessively. Some individuals may experience side effects, including digestive discomfort or headaches. Using horsetail species intended for consumption is critical, as some species can contain toxic compounds. Consult with a healthcare provider before using horsetail for specific health concerns, especially if you have underlying health conditions or are taking medications. Horsetail is a plant with potential health benefits, particularly concerning its diuretic properties and use in promoting skin and hair health. It should be used cautiously and under the guidance of a qualified herbalist or healthcare provider, especially if you are taking medications or have underlying health conditions. Always seek professional advice before using horsetail as a natural remedy.

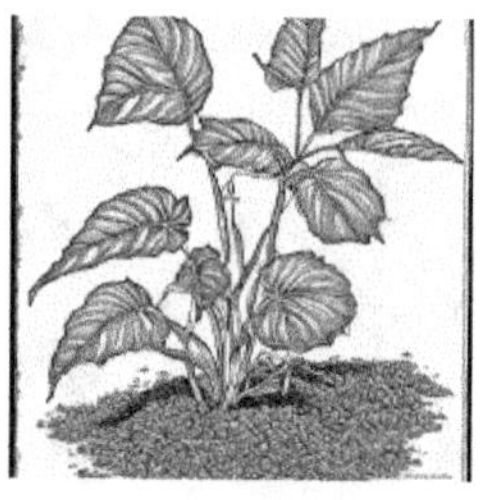

Kava (Piper methysticum) is a plant native to the South Pacific, particularly in regions like Fiji, Tonga, and Vanuatu. It is well-known for its use in traditional Pacific Island cultures as a ceremonial beverage and for its potential medicinal properties. Here is a detailed overview of kava, including its historical use, preparation, medicinal properties, visual identification, precautions, and potential health benefits.

Historical Use: Kava has a long history of use in the South Pacific, where it is consumed in social and ceremonial contexts. It is used for its calming and sedative effects and is believed to promote relaxation and a sense of well-being.

Preparation: To prepare kava, the kava plant's roots are traditionally harvested. The roots are dug up, cleaned, and peeled.
Macerated: The peeled roots are pounded or grated into a pulp. Mixed with Water: The kava pulp is mixed with water, and the liquid is extracted. Filtered: The liquid is strained to remove solid particles. Consumed: The resulting kava beverage is consumed in a social setting.

Medicinal Properties: Kava is traditionally used for its potential health benefits, including Relaxation. Kava is known for its calming and anxiolytic (anxiety reducing) effects. Sleep Aid: It may help improve sleep and alleviate insomnia. Muscle Relaxant: Kava may act as a muscle relaxant, helping to reduce tension and muscle pain. Anti-Inflammatory: It is believed to have anti-inflammatory properties and may help reduce inflammation and pain.

Visual Identification: Kava plants can be recognized by the following characteristics: Large, heart-shaped leaves. Spiky, spherical flower clusters. Thick, tuberous roots that are used to make kava.

Precautions:
While kava has been traditionally consumed in the South Pacific for centuries, concerns have been raised about its potential impact on the liver. Some individuals have reported liver toxicity associated with kava consumption. Using kava supplements or extracts has raised safety concerns and regulatory restrictions in some countries. Individuals with a history of liver problems, heavy alcohol use, or those taking medications that affect the liver should avoid kava. Consult with a healthcare provider before using kava for specific health concerns, especially if you have underlying health conditions or are taking medications.

Kava is a traditional South Pacific beverage known for its potential relaxation and calming effects. It is used in social and ceremonial contexts and is valued for its cultural significance. However, it should be used with caution, especially in supplement form, and under the guidance of a qualified healthcare provider. If you are considering using kava for its potential health benefits, consult a healthcare provider to discuss any potential risks and benefits.

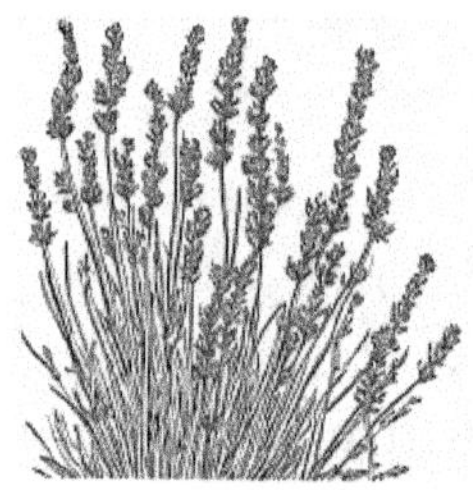

Lavender (Lavandula angustifolia) is a fragrant herb and a popular plant known for its aromatic flowers and potential medicinal properties. It has been used for centuries in traditional medicine and various other purposes. Here is a detailed overview of lavender, including its historical use, cultivation, visual identification, medicinal properties, precautions, and potential health benefits.

Historical Use: Lavender has a long history of use, dating back to ancient civilizations. It has been used in several ways, including for its fragrance, medicinal properties, and in herbal remedies.

Cultivation: Lavender is a hardy, perennial plant that is easy to grow. It is cultivated in gardens and used for its fragrant flowers. Lavender typically prefers well-drained soil and plenty of sunlight.

Visual Identification: Lavender plants can be recognized by the following characteristics: Fragrant, slender spikes of small, tubular flowers in shades of purple, blue, pink, or white. Silver-gray or green leaves that are narrow and lance shaped. Lavender bushes are typically compact and grow to varying heights depending on the variety. Medicinal Properties: Lavender is traditionally used for potential health benefits, including Relaxation. It is known for its calming and relaxing properties and is often used in aromatherapy to reduce stress and anxiety. Sleep Aid: It may help improve sleep quality and reduce insomnia. Pain Relief: Lavender essential oil may be used topically to relieve minor pain and discomfort. Skin Care: Lavender essential oil is applied to the skin to soothe minor burns, insect bites, and skin irritations. Antioxidant: Lavender contains antioxidants that help protect cells from oxidative stress.

Precautions: Lavender is considered safe for most people when used in moderation. However, some individuals may experience skin irritation or allergies when using lavender essential oil. If you plan to use lavender essential oil on your skin, it is crucial to dilute it with carrier oil and perform a patch test to check for sensitivity. While lavender is safe for many, consult a healthcare provider before using it, especially if you are pregnant, breastfeeding, or have underlying health conditions.

Lavender is a beloved herb known for its fragrance and potential health benefits, particularly relaxation, sleep, and skincare. It is safe to use in moderation, and lavender essential oil is popular for aromatherapy and skin applications. However, always use caution when using essential oils and consult with a healthcare provider before using lavender for specific health concerns, especially if you have underlying health conditions or are pregnant or breastfeeding.

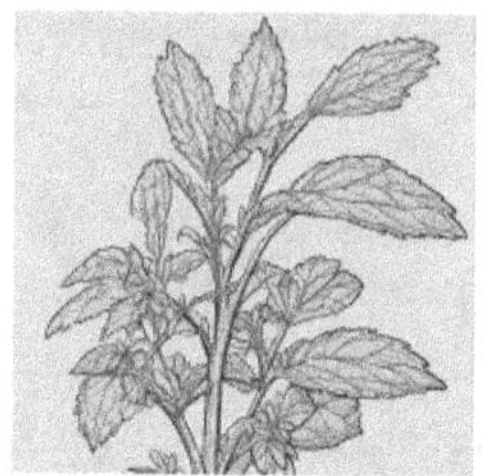 **Lemon balm (Melissa officinalis)** is a fragrant herb in the mint family, known for its pleasant lemony aroma and potential medicinal properties. It has been used for centuries in traditional herbal medicine and as a culinary herb. Here is a detailed overview of lemon balm, including its historical use, cultivation, visual identification, medicinal properties, precautions, and potential health benefits.

Historical Use: Lemon balm has a long history of use in traditional medicine, dating back to ancient Greece and Rome. It was valued for its potential calming and soothing effects.

Cultivation:
Lemon balm is a hardy, perennial herb that is easy to grow. It is cultivated in gardens and used for its aromatic leaves. Lemon balm typically prefers well-drained soil and partial shade but can tolerate full sun.

Visual Identification: Lemon balm plants can be recognized by the following characteristics: Bright green, heart-shaped leaves with serrated edges. Small, white, or pale pink flowers that grow in clusters. A distinctive lemon fragrance when the leaves are crushed.

Medicinal Properties: Lemon balm is traditionally used for potential health benefits, including relaxation. Lemon balm is known for its calming and stress-reducing properties and is often used to alleviate anxiety and promote relaxation.

Sleep Aid: It may help improve sleep quality and reduce insomnia. Digestive Health: Lemon balm is used to ease digestive issues like indigestion and gas. Antioxidant: Lemon balm contains antioxidants that help protect cells from oxidative stress. Topical Use: It can be applied topically to soothe cold sores and insect bites.

Precautions: Lemon balm is considered safe when used in moderation. However, some individuals may experience mild side effects like gastrointestinal discomfort. While lemon balm is safe for most people, consult a healthcare provider before using it, especially if you are pregnant, breastfeeding, or have underlying health conditions. Lemon balm is a popular herb known for its pleasant, lemony fragrance and potential health benefits, particularly with relaxation, sleep, and digestive health. It is widely used in teas and herbal preparations and is safe to use in moderation. Consult with a healthcare provider before using lemon balm for specific health concerns, especially if you have underlying health conditions or are pregnant or breastfeeding.

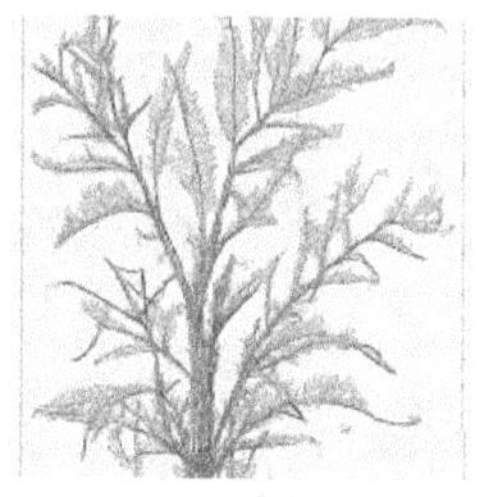

Licorice (Glycyrrhiza glabra) is a well-known herb with a distinct sweet flavor and a long history of use in traditional medicine and as a flavoring agent. It is native to parts of Europe and Asia and is known for its potential medicinal properties. Here is a detailed overview of licorice, including its historical use, visual identification, medicinal properties, growth conditions, cultivation, precautions, and potential health benefits.

Historical Use: Licorice has been used for thousands of years in various traditional medicine systems, including Ayurveda, Traditional Chinese Medicine (TCM), and Western herbalism. It was valued for its potential health benefits and sweet flavor.

Visual Identification: Licorice plants can be recognized by the following characteristics: Compound leaves with numerous leaflets. Small, bluish-purple, or whitish-pink flowers that grow in spikes.

A deep taproot that is used in herbal preparations. Medicinal Properties: Licorice is traditionally used for potential health benefits, including Sore Throat and Cough. Licorice is known for its soothing properties and often relieves sore throats and coughs. Anti-Inflammatory: It is believed to have anti-inflammatory properties that can help reduce inflammation and pain.

Digestive Health: Licorice is used to alleviate digestive issues, such as indigestion and heartburn. Adrenal Support: Licorice may support the adrenal glands and hormone regulation, particularly in traditional Chinese medicine. Antioxidant: It

350

contains antioxidants that help protect cells from oxidative stress.

Growth Conditions: Licorice prefers specific conditions for optimal growth: Well-drained soil, particularly sandy or loamy soil.
Full sun or partial shade. A warm, temperate climate.

Cultivation:
Licorice can be grown from seeds or root cuttings. It is a perennial plant and may take a few years to establish and produce a
harvestable root. The roots are typically harvested in the fall.

Precautions:
Licorice is considered safe when used in moderation but should not be consumed excessively. Licorice consumption can lead to side effects, including high blood pressure and potassium imbalance. Individuals with certain health conditions, such as high blood pressure, should avoid licorice or use it with caution. Consult with a healthcare provider before using licorice for specific health concerns, especially if you have underlying health conditions or are taking medications.

Licorice is a versatile herb known for its potential health benefits, particularly in relation to soothing sore throats, relieving coughs, and supporting digestive health. It is widely used in teas and herbal preparations and is safe to use in moderation. However, individuals with certain health conditions should exercise caution. Consult with a healthcare provider before using licorice for specific health concerns, especially if you have underlying health conditions or are taking medications.

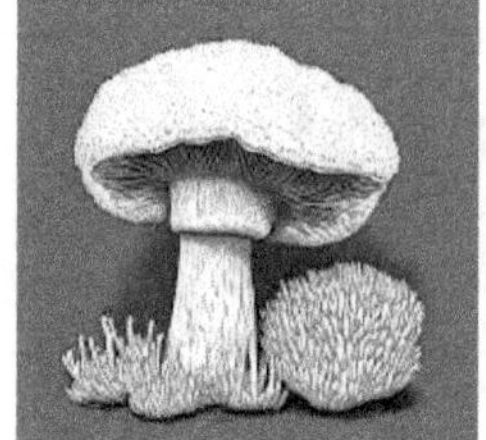

Lion's Mane Mushroom (Hericium erinaceus) is a unique and edible mushroom with potential medicinal properties. It is known for its distinctive appearance and health benefits. Here is a detailed overview of Lion's Mane Mushroom, including its historical use, visual identification, medicinal properties, growth conditions, cultivation, precautions, and potential health benefits.

Historical Use: Lion's Mane Mushroom has been used in traditional Chinese and Japanese medicine for centuries. It was traditionally believed to support cognitive function and overall health.

Visual Identification: Lion's Mane Mushroom can be recognized by the following characteristics: White, cascading, and elongated spines that resemble a lion's mane. No traditional cap and stem like many other mushrooms. A mild, seafood-like aroma and taste when cooked.

Medicinal Properties: Lion's Mane Mushroom is traditionally used for its potential health benefits, including Cognitive Support. It is believed to have neuroprotective properties and may support cognitive function and memory. Nerve Regeneration: Lion's Mane is thought to stimulate nerve growth factors and promote the regeneration of nerve cells. Immune Support: It may help strengthen the immune system. Anti-Inflammatory: It is believed to have anti-inflammatory properties that can help reduce inflammation and pain.

Growth Conditions: Lion's Mane Mushroom is a wood-loving fungus and is often found growing on hardwood trees, particularly oak and beech. It prefers a temperate climate in North America, Europe, and Asia.

Cultivation: Lion's Mane Mushroom can be cultivated on hardwood logs or sawdust substrate. Cultivating it at home or in a controlled environment is possible using Lion's Mane Mushroom grow kits.

Precautions: Lion's Mane Mushroom is considered safe when consumed as food or in supplement form. While no known significant side effects exist, some individuals may experience mild digestive discomfort. If you have allergies to mushrooms or fungi, exercise caution when trying Lion's Mane. Consult with a healthcare provider before using Lion's Mane supplements for specific health concerns, especially if you have underlying health conditions.

Lion's Mane Mushroom is a fascinating fungus known for its potential health benefits, particularly in relation to cognitive support, nerve regeneration, and immune health. It is commonly used in culinary dishes and can also be consumed in supplement form. Consult with a healthcare provider before using Lion's Mane for specific health concerns, especially if you have underlying health conditions.

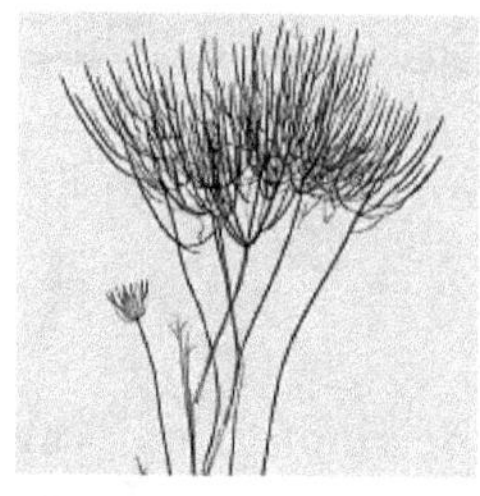

Lomatium (Lomatium dissectum), also known as desert parsley, is a flowering plant native to North America. It is recognized for its traditional medicinal uses, particularly among Indigenous communities in the western United States.

Lomatium has potential therapeutic properties, and it has gained attention for its possible immune-supporting effects. Here is a detailed overview of Lomatium, including its historical use, visual identification, medicinal properties, growth conditions, precautions, and potential health benefits.

Historical Use: Lomatium has a long history of use among Indigenous peoples in North America. Various tribes have traditionally used it for its potential medicinal properties, such as treating respiratory ailments and infections and supporting overall health.

Visual Identification: Lomatium plants can be recognized by the following characteristics: Umbels of small, yellow flowers. Pinnately compound leaves with numerous leaflets. Long, slender stems with a characteristic parsley-like appearance.

Medicinal Properties. Lomatium is traditionally used for its potential health benefits, including Immune Support. Lomatium is believed to support the immune system and may have antiviral and antimicrobial properties. Respiratory Health: It has been used to alleviate respiratory issues, including coughs, colds, and bronchial infections. Anti-Inflammatory: Lomatium is thought to have anti-inflammatory properties that can help reduce inflammation and pain.

Growth Conditions: Lomatium is typically found in arid and semi-arid regions of western North America, including parts of California, Nevada, and the Great Basin. It thrives in well-drained soil and is often found in desert and sagebrush ecosystems.

Cultivation: Cultivating Lomatium typically involves growing it from seeds. It can be challenging to cultivate outside of its natural habitat, as it has specific growth requirements and may take several years to mature.

Precautions: While Lomatium has a history of safe traditional use, it is essential to exercise caution when using it in any form, especially in concentrated extracts or supplements. Some individuals may experience allergic reactions or skin sensitivities when handling Lomatium. Consult with a healthcare provider before using Lomatium for specific health concerns, especially if you have underlying health conditions or are taking medications. Lomatium is a plant recognized for its potential immune-supporting and respiratory health benefits. It is traditionally used in herbal preparations and may be available in various forms, such as tinctures or capsules. If you are considering using Lomatium for its potential health benefits, consult with a healthcare provider before use, especially if you have underlying health conditions or are taking medications.

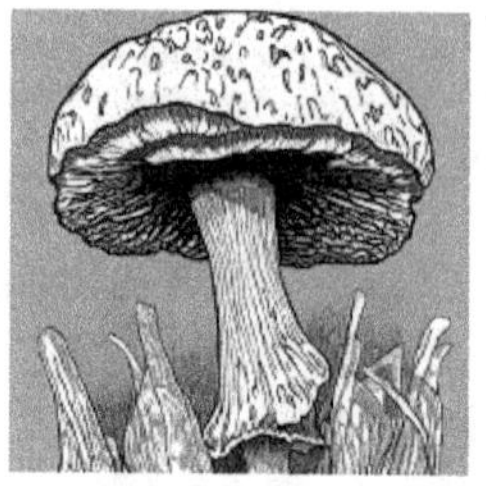

Maitake Mushroom (Grifola frondosa) is a type of edible mushroom with potential medicinal properties. It is commonly found in North America and Asia and has been used for centuries in traditional medicine. Maitake is known for its potential health benefits, particularly concerning immune support and overall wellness. Here is a detailed overview of Maitake Mushroom, including its historical use, visual identification, medicinal properties, growth conditions, cultivation, precautions, and potential health benefits.

Historical Use: Maitake mushrooms have been used for their potential medicinal properties in traditional Chinese and Japanese medicine for centuries. They were traditionally valued for their potential immune-supporting effects.

Visual Identification: Maitake mushrooms can be recognized by the following characteristics: A large, cluster-like appearance with multiple fan-shaped caps. Gray-brown or brownish colors. The individual caps have a layered or wrinkled appearance.

Medicinal Properties: Maitake is traditionally used for its potential health benefits, including immune support. Maitake mushrooms are believed to support the immune system and may have antiviral and antimicrobial properties. Anti-Inflammatory: It is thought to have anti-inflammatory properties that can help reduce inflammation and pain. Blood Sugar Control: Some studies suggest that Maitake may help regulate blood sugar levels.

Adaptogenic: It is considered an adaptogenic herb, which may help the body adapt to stress and maintain overall wellness.

Growth: Maitake mushrooms are typically found in hardwood forests and are known to grow in association with the base of oak, maple, and elm trees. They thrive in temperate regions and can be found in parts of North America, Europe, and Asia.

Cultivation: Cultivating Maitake mushrooms typically involve growing them on hardwood logs or sawdust substrate. It is possible to cultivate Maitake mushrooms at home is possible using Maitake mushroom grow kits.

Precautions: Maitake mushrooms are considered safe when consumed as food or in supplement form. However, it is essential to purchase them from reputable sources. If you are allergic to mushrooms or fungi, exercise caution when trying Maitake.
Consult with a healthcare provider before using Maitake supplements for specific health concerns, especially if you have underlying health conditions or are taking medications.

Maitake mushrooms are a valued edible and medicinal mushroom known for their potential immune-supporting and anti-inflammatory properties. They are commonly used in culinary dishes and are available in supplement form. Consult with a healthcare provider before using Maitake for specific health concerns, especially if you have underlying health conditions or are taking medications.

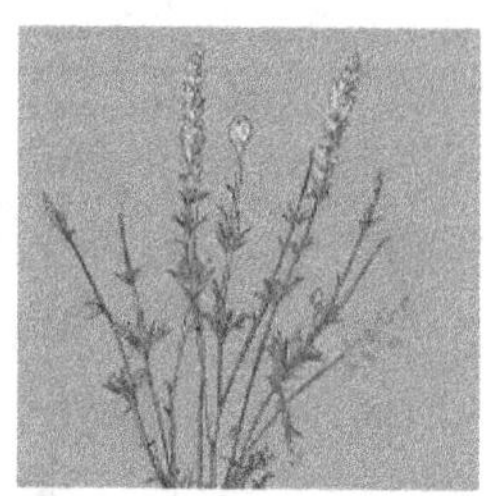

Marshmallow (Althaea officinalis) is a perennial herb with a long history of use in traditional medicine, dating back to ancient civilizations. It is known for its potential medicinal properties, particularly its soothing effects on the respiratory and digestive systems. Here is a detailed overview of marshmallow, including its historical use, visual identification, medicinal properties, growth conditions, cultivation, precautions, and potential health benefits:

Historical Use: Marshmallow has a history of use that spans thousands of years. It was used benefits and culinary purposes. In traditional medicine, it was valued for its soothing properties.

Visual Identification: Marshmallow plants can be recognized by the following characteristics: Tall, upright stems with serrated leaves. Pink or pale purple flowers with five petals. The roots are particularly valued for their mucilaginous properties.

Medicinal Properties. Marshmallow is traditionally used for its potential health benefits, including Respiratory Health. It is known for its soothing effects on the respiratory system, particularly in alleviating coughs and sore throats. Digestive Health: Marshmallow is used to soothe the digestive tract and relieve issues like heartburn, gastritis, and irritable bowel syndrome. Skin Health: It may be applied topically to soothe skin irritations and minor wounds. Anti-Inflammatory: Marshmallow is believed to have anti-inflammatory properties that can help reduce inflammation and pain.

Growth Conditions: Marshmallow is typically found in wetlands and along the edges of rivers and ponds. It thrives in moist, well-drained soil and is native to parts of Europe and Asia.

Cultivation: Cultivating marshmallow typically involves growing it from seeds or root cuttings. It is a hardy plant and can be grown in gardens under the right conditions.

Precautions: Marshmallows are considered safe when used as directed but should not be consumed excessively. If you have allergies to plants in the Malvaceae family (which includes marshmallow), you may be sensitive to marshmallow. Consult with a healthcare provider before using marshmallow supplements or extracts for specific health concerns, especially if you have underlying health conditions or are taking medications.

Marshmallow is a versatile herb known for its potential soothing effects on the respiratory and digestive systems. It is widely used in teas and herbal preparations and is safe to use in moderation. Consult with a healthcare provider before using marshmallow for specific health concerns, especially if you have underlying health conditions or are taking medications.

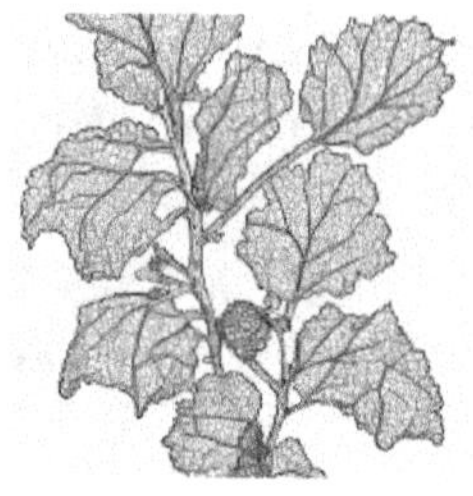 **Mulberries (Morus spp.)** are deciduous trees or shrubs known for their sweet and juicy fruits. These fruits are not only delicious but also have potential health benefits. Here is a detailed overview of mulberries, including their historical use, visual identification, growth conditions, cultivation, medicinal properties, precautions, and potential health benefits.

Historical Use: Mulberries have been cultivated for their fruits for thousands of years, with a history that spans several cultures, including those in Asia, Europe, and the Middle East. They have been used for their sweet taste and as a traditional remedy for various health issues.

Visual Identification: Mulberry trees or shrubs can be recognized by the following characteristics: Simple, alternate leaves that are often lobed or serrated. Small, sweet, and multiple fruit clusters that can be red, white, or black in color, depending on the variety.

Growth Conditions: Mulberry trees are hardy and can grow in various soil types. They prefer well-drained soil and full sun. Mulberries are commonly grown in many regions, and distinct species have adapted to various climates.

Cultivation: Mulberries can be cultivated from seeds, cuttings, or grafted plants. They are low-maintenance and can be grown in gardens and orchards. Pruning and maintenance are necessary to control their size and shape.

Medicinal Properties: Mulberries are traditionally used for their potential health benefits, including Antioxidant Properties. Mulberries are rich in anthocyanins, resveratrol, and vitamin C, making them a source of antioxidants that help protect cells from oxidative damage. Blood Sugar Control: Some studies suggest that mulberries may help regulate blood sugar levels. Heart Health: The antioxidants in mulberries may support cardiovascular health by reducing inflammation and promoting healthy blood vessels. Digestive Health: The high fiber content in mulberries can support digestive health and regularity. Precautions:

Mulberries are considered safe when consumed as food or in moderate amounts. However, some individuals may experience digestive discomfort if consumed excessively. If you have allergies to plants in the Moraceae family (which includes mulberries), you may be sensitive to mulberries. Consult with a healthcare provider before using mulberry supplements or extracts for specific health concerns, especially if you have underlying health conditions or are taking medications.

Mulberries are delicious fruits with potential health benefits, particularly concerning their antioxidant properties and potential effects on blood sugar and heart health. They are commonly enjoyed fresh, dried, or in culinary dishes and jams. Consult with a healthcare provider before using mulberries for specific health concerns, especially if you have underlying health conditions or are taking medications.

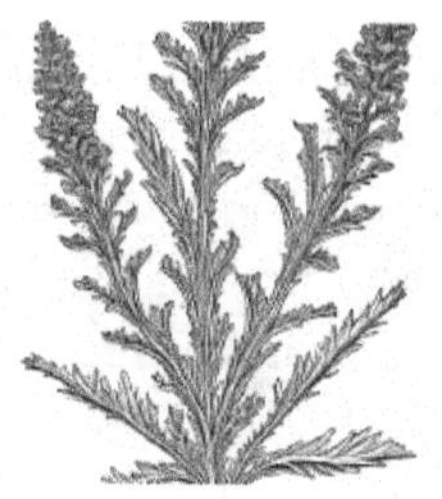

Mullein (Verbascum thapsus)

is a biennial plant native to Europe but has naturalized in many parts of the world, including North America. It has a long history of use in traditional herbal medicine and is known for its potential medicinal properties. Here is a detailed overview of mullein, including its historical use, visual identification, growth conditions, cultivation, medicinal properties, precautions, and potential health benefits.

Historical Use: Mullein has a history of use in traditional herbal medicine that dates back hundreds of years. Various parts of the plant, including the leaves and flowers, have been used to make herbal remedies for respiratory and other health issues.

Visual Identification: The following characteristics can recognize mullein plants: A tall, biennial plant with a rosette of large, fuzzy leaves in the first year. In the second year, it produces a tall flowering stalk with yellow, densely packed flowers. The leaves and flowers are covered in soft, downy hairs.

Growth Conditions: Mullein prefers well-drained soil and is often found in disturbed areas, along roadsides, and in fields. It can thrive in various soil types and is drought tolerant.

Cultivation: Mullein can be cultivated in gardens and is typically grown from seeds. It is easy to grow and does not require extensive care.

Medicinal Properties: Mullein is traditionally used for its potential health benefits, including Respiratory Health. It is known for its soothing effects on the respiratory system and is often used to alleviate coughs, bronchitis, and other respiratory issues.

Anti-Inflammatory: Mullein is believed to have anti-inflammatory properties that can help reduce inflammation and pain.
Ear Health: The infused oil from mullein flowers has been used in herbal ear drops to alleviate earaches. Expectorant: It may help to loosen and expel mucus from the respiratory tract.

Precautions: Mullein is considered safe when used as directed. However, the plant can cause skin irritation in some individuals due to the fine hairs on the leaves. If you are allergic to plants in the Scrophulariaceae family (which includes mullein), you may be sensitive to mullein. Consult with a healthcare provider before using mullein supplements or extracts for specific health concerns, especially if you have underlying health conditions or are taking medications.

Mullein is a versatile herb known for its potential soothing effects on the respiratory system and various medicinal properties. It is commonly used in herbal preparations such as teas and tinctures. Consult with a healthcare provider before using mullein for specific health concerns, especially if you have underlying health conditions or are taking medications.

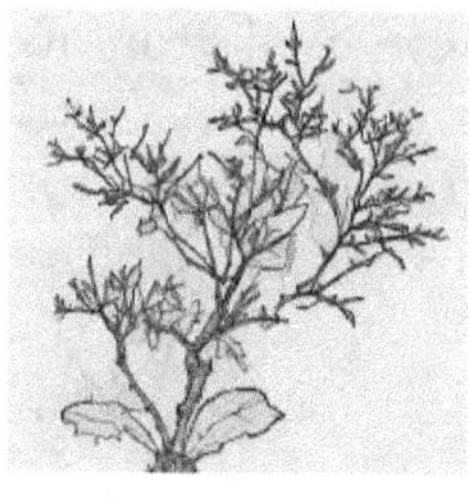

Myrrh (Commiphora myrrha)

is a resin obtained from the bark of small, thorny myrrh trees native to the Arabian Peninsula and parts of East Africa. Myrrh has a long history of use in traditional medicine, religious rituals, and perfumery. It is known for its potential medicinal properties and various applications. Here is a detailed overview of myrrh, including its historical use, visual identification, growth conditions, cultivation, medicinal properties, precautions, and potential health benefits.

Historical Use: Myrrh has a rich history dating back thousands of years. It was highly valued in ancient Egypt, Greece, and the Middle East for its use in religious rituals, embalming, and traditional medicine. Traditional Chinese and Ayurvedic medicine were used for its potential health benefits.

Visual Identification: Myrrh is obtained from small, thorny myrrh trees, which have the following characteristics can identify:
Small, knotty tree with a bushy appearance. Pinnately compound leaves with multiple leaflets. Resin is harvested from the tree's bark and appears as dry, amber to reddish-brown tears.

Growth Conditions: Myrrh trees thrive in arid and semi-arid regions with well-drained soil. They are drought-resistant and can tolerate harsh environmental conditions.

Cultivation: Cultivating myrrh trees can be challenging due to their specific growth requirements and slow growth rate. They can be propagated from seeds, but the trees may take several years to reach maturity.

Medicinal Properties: Myrrh is traditionally used for its potential health benefits, including Anti-Inflammatory: Myrrh is believed to have anti-inflammatory properties that can help reduce inflammation and pain. Antimicrobial: It has been used for its potential antimicrobial and antibacterial properties. Oral Health: Myrrh has been used in oral care products for its potential to promote healthy gums and relieve mouth irritations. Wound Healing: It may promote wound healing and reduce the risk of infection. Respiratory Health: Myrrh is known for its soothing effects on the respiratory system and is often used to alleviate coughs and bronchial issues.

Precautions: Myrrh is considered safe when used as directed. However, it may cause skin irritation in some individuals when applied topically. Consult with a healthcare provider before using myrrh supplements or extracts for specific health concerns, especially if you have underlying health conditions or are taking medications.

Myrrh is a resin with a rich history and a wide range of potential medicinal applications. It is used in various forms, including essential oils, tinctures, and topical products. Consult with a healthcare provider before using myrrh for specific health concerns, especially if you have underlying health conditions or are taking medications.

N-acetylcysteine (NAC) is a medication and dietary supplement that is a modified form of the amino acid cysteine. It is known for its potential medicinal properties and is used for various health-related purposes. Here is a detailed overview of N-acetylcysteine (NAC), including its uses, dosage, precautions, and potential health benefits.

Uses: NAC has a range of potential uses, including Respiratory Health. NAC is commonly used as a mucolytic agent to help break down and thin mucus, making it easier to clear from the airways. It is often used in treating chronic respiratory conditions such as chronic obstructive pulmonary disease (COPD), asthma, and cystic fibrosis. It may also be used as an antidote in cases of acetaminophen (paracetamol) overdose cases. Psychiatric Disorders: Some studies suggest that NAC may have potential benefits for mental health conditions such as obsessive-compulsive disorder (OCD), depression, and bipolar disorder. It is believed to work by modulating glutamate levels and reducing oxidative stress.

Antioxidant Properties: NAC is known for its antioxidant properties and can help protect cells from oxidative damage. This makes it a potential adjunct in various health conditions related to oxidative stress. Liver Health: NAC may support liver health and detoxification processes. Bronchitis and COPD: NAC is used to alleviate symptoms of chronic bronchitis and COPD, such as cough and mucus production.

Dosage: The appropriate dosage of NAC can vary depending on the specific health condition and individual needs. Dosages typically range from 600 mg to 1,800 mg per day, but higher doses may be recommended for certain conditions. It is crucial to follow the dosing instructions provided on the product label or as directed by a healthcare provider.

Precautions: NAC is considered safe when used as directed. However, some individuals may experience side effects like gastrointestinal discomfort or skin rashes. If you are pregnant, breastfeeding, have underlying health conditions, or are taking medications, consult with a healthcare provider before using NAC.

NAC is a versatile supplement with various potential health benefits, particularly in relation to respiratory health, mental health, and antioxidant support. It is commonly available in dietary supplement form and is used under a healthcare provider's guidance to address health concerns. Always follow the dosing instructions provided on the product label or as directed by a healthcare provider.

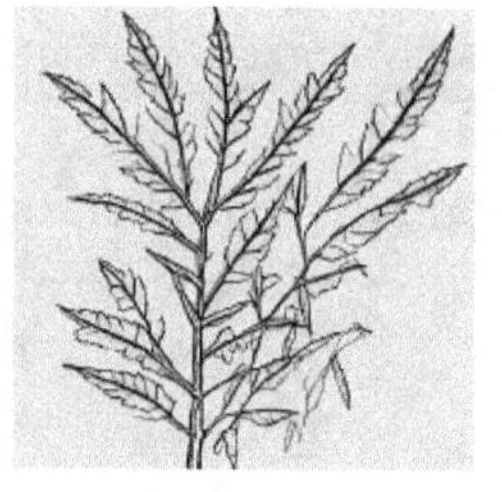

Neem (Azadirachta indica) is a tree native to the Indian subcontinent and known for its many traditional and medicinal uses. Neem is often called the "wonder tree" because of its wide range of applications, particularly in traditional Ayurvedic and other herbal systems of medicine. Here is a detailed overview of neem, including its historical use, visual identification, growth conditions, cultivation, medicinal properties, precautions, and potential health benefits.

Historical Use: Neem has a long history of use in traditional medicine, particularly in Ayurveda, where it is considered a powerful medicinal plant. It is used for various purposes, including skincare, haircare, and the treatment of a wide range of health conditions,

Visual Identification: Neem trees can be recognized by the following characteristics: Evergreen is a fast-growing tree with compound leaves containing 10-31 leaflets. Small, fragrant white flowers. Yellow to green, ellipsoidal fruits with a single seed inside.

Growth Conditions: Neem trees thrive in regions with tropical and subtropical climates. They are drought-resistant and can tolerate a wide range of soil types. Neem is often found in parts of India, Southeast Asia, and Africa.

Cultivation: Neem trees can be cultivated from seeds and require well-drained soil. They are low-maintenance and can grow in gardens, orchards, and windbreaks.

Medicinal Properties: Neem is traditionally used for its potential health benefits, including antimicrobial: Neem has strong antimicrobial properties and is used for skin conditions, wounds, and infections. Skin Health: It is used for treating skin conditions like acne, eczema, and psoriasis. Oral Health: Neem is used in oral care products for its potential to promote healthy gums and teeth. Antioxidant: Neem is rich in antioxidants that help protect cells from oxidative damage. Anti-Inflammatory: It is believed to have anti-inflammatory properties that can help reduce inflammation and pain.

Precautions: Neem is considered safe when used externally for skin care and oral care. However, it may cause skin irritation or allergic reactions in some individuals. Neem oil should not be ingested, as it may have toxic effects. Consult with a healthcare provider before using neem supplements or extracts for specific health concerns, especially if you have underlying health conditions or are taking medications.

Neem is a versatile plant known for its potential medicinal properties, particularly in relation to skincare, oral health, and overall well-being. It is commonly used in various forms, including neem oil, leaves, and neem extracts. Consult with a healthcare provider before using neem for specific health concerns, especially if you have underlying health conditions or are taking medications.

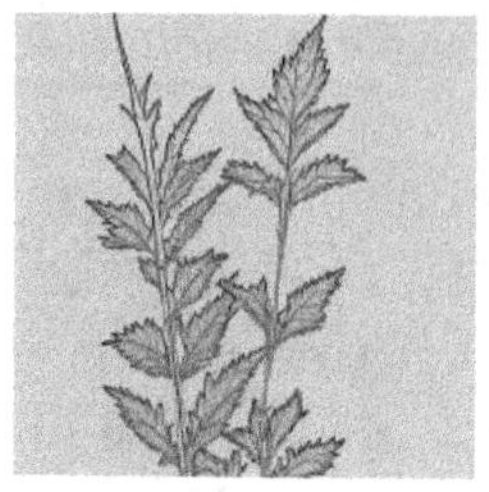**Nettle (Urtica dioica)** is a common flowering plant with a long history of use in traditional medicine and as a food source. It is known for its potential medicinal properties and is used to treat various health issues. Here is a detailed overview of nettle, including its historical use, visual identification, growth conditions, cultivation, medicinal properties, precautions, and potential health benefits.

Historical Use: Nettle has a history of use in traditional medicine, dating back to ancient times. Various cultures have used nettle for its medicinal and culinary properties, primarily for its potential to alleviate conditions related to allergies and inflammation.

Visual Identification: Nettle plants can be recognized by the following characteristics: Coarsely toothed opposite leaves with serrated edges. Stinging hairs (trichomes) on the leaves and stems can cause skin irritation upon contact. Small, greenish, or whitish flowers in clusters.

Growth Conditions: Nettle is a hardy, perennial plant that can be found in temperate regions throughout the world. It often grows in moist and nitrogen-rich soil, along stream banks, and in woodlands.

Cultivation: Nettle can be cultivated from seeds or propagated by dividing established plants. It is easy to grow and can be planted in gardens or as part of a naturalized landscape.

Medicinal Properties: Nettle is traditionally used for its potential health benefits, including Anti-Inflammatory: Nettle is believed to have anti-inflammatory properties that can help reduce inflammation and pain. Allergy Relief: It is used to alleviate symptoms of allergies, such as hay fever and allergic rhinitis. Diuretic: Nettle may have diuretic properties and promote healthy urine flow. Nutrient-Rich: Nettle leaves are a source of vitamins and minerals, particularly vitamins A and C, iron, and calcium.

Precautions: The stinging hairs on nettle plants can cause skin irritation upon contact, so it is advisable to wear gloves when handling them. When consumed as a food or supplement, nettles are considered safe. However, if you are pregnant, breastfeeding, have underlying health conditions, or are taking medications, consult a healthcare provider before using nettle for specific health concerns.

Nettle is a versatile plant known for its potential health benefits, particularly in relation to allergy relief and anti-inflammatory properties. It is commonly consumed as tea, used in culinary dishes, or taken in supplement form. Consult with a healthcare provider before using Nettle for specific health concerns, especially if you have underlying health conditions or are taking medications.

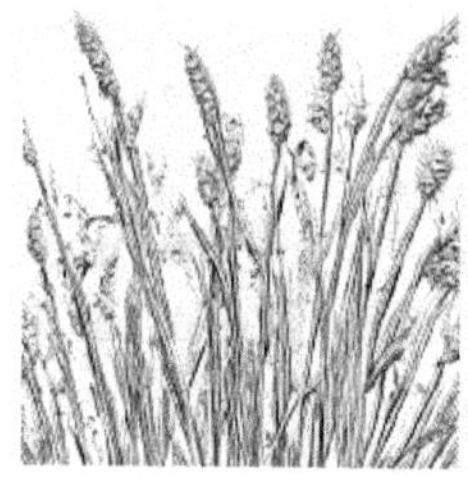

Oats (Avena sativa) are a widely cultivated cereal grain known for their nutritional value and various culinary and medicinal uses. Oats are a staple food in many parts of the world and are recognized for their potential health benefits. Here is a detailed overview of oats, including their historical use, visual identification, growth conditions, cultivation, nutritional properties, culinary uses, and potential health benefits.

Historical Use: Oats have a long history of cultivation and use, dating back to ancient civilizations. They have been consumed as a food source and used for their potential health benefits.

Visual Identification: Oat plants can be recognized by the following characteristics: Grass-like, upright plants with hollow stems. Long, linear leaves and a loose cluster of small, inconspicuous flowers. Oat grains, commonly referred to as oat groats, are the seeds of the plant and are typically hulled for consumption.

Growth Conditions: Oats thrive in temperate climates and are commonly grown in regions with cool, moist conditions. They are often cultivated as a winter crop in areas where they can withstand frost.

Cultivation: Oats are typically grown from seeds and can be cultivated in gardens or on a larger scale as a field crop. They are known for their adaptability and can tolerate a range of soil types.

Nutritional Properties: Oats are highly nutritious and a good Dietary Fiber source. Oats are rich in soluble fiber, particularly beta-glucans, which are known to support heart health and help regulate blood sugar levels. Protein: Oats contain a moderate amount of protein. Complex Carbohydrates: They provide a steady source of energy. Vitamins and Minerals: Oats are a source of vitamins, such as B vitamins, and minerals like manganese, phosphorus, and magnesium.

Culinary Uses: Oats are used in various culinary applications, including oatmeal, granola, and muesli, as an ingredient in baked goods like cookies and bread. Oatmeal is commonly consumed as a hot breakfast cereal, and oats are a versatile ingredient in many   recipes.

Potential Health Benefits: Oats are recognized for their potential health benefits, including Heart Health: The beta-glucans in oats have been linked to reduced cholesterol levels and improved heart health. Blood Sugar Control: Oats may help regulate blood sugar levels due to their high fiber content. Digestive Health: Oats can support digestive health due to their fiber content. Weight Management: The fiber in oats helps promote a feeling of fullness, making them a valuable food for weight management.

Oats are a nutritious grain known for their versatility and potential health benefits. They are commonly consumed as a wholesome and healthy food source. If you have dietary concerns or health conditions, consult with a healthcare provider or a registered dietitian for personalized guidance on incorporating oats.

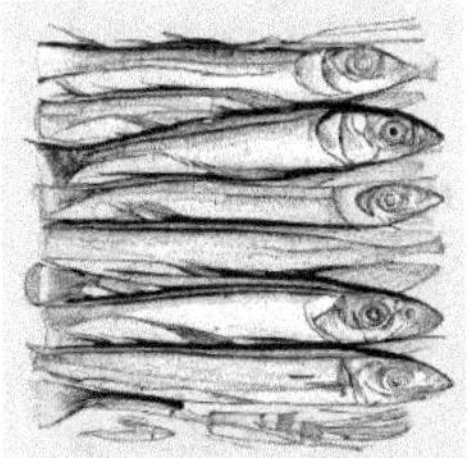

Omega-3 fatty acids are a group of essential polyunsaturated fats that are important for overall health. There are three primary omega-3 fatty acids that are commonly found in fish and seafood: Eicosapentaenoic Acid (EPA), EPA is known for its anti-inflammatory properties and is associated with cardiovascular health. It is commonly found in fatty fish such as salmon, mackerel, and sardines. Docosahexaenoic Acid (DHA): DHA is crucial for brain health, especially during pregnancy and infancy. It is found in high concentrations in fatty fish and seafood and in fish oil supplements. Alpha-Linolenic Acid (ALA): ALA is found in plant sources like flaxseeds, chia seeds, and walnuts. It can be converted into EPA and DHA in the body, but the conversion is limited.

Here is a detailed overview of omega-3 fatty acids from fish, including their sources, nutritional properties, health benefits, precautions, and potential uses.

Sources: Omega-3 fatty acids, particularly EPA and DHA, are found in several types of fish and seafood, including salmon, mackerel, sardines, trout, herring, tuna, and anchovies.

Nutritional Properties: Omega-3 fatty acids have several critical nutritional properties: Anti-Inflammatory: They have anti-inflammatory properties that may reduce the risk of chronic diseases.

Heart Health: Omega-3s are associated with improved heart health by reducing the risk of heart disease, lowering triglycerides, and improving cholesterol levels.

Brain Health: DHA, in particular, is essential for brain health, especially during development and in maintaining cognitive function. Eye Health: Omega-3s may support eye health and reduce the risk of age-related macular degeneration.

Potential Health Benefits: Omega-3 fatty acids from fish are associated with many potential health benefits, including Reduced Inflammation. They can help reduce inflammation in the body, which is linked to various chronic diseases. Cardiovascular Health: Omega-3s may reduce the risk of heart disease by improving blood lipid profiles and reducing blood pressure. Brain Function: DHA is critical in brain development and may help support adult cognitive function. Eye Health: Omega-3s may help reduce the risk of age-related macular degeneration, a common cause of vision loss in older adults.

Precautions: While omega-3 fatty acids from fish are considered safe and beneficial for most people, they can interact with blood-thinning medications like warfarin, so it is essential to consult with a healthcare provider if you are taking such medications. Some individuals may be allergic to fish, and fish oil supplements should be used with caution in such cases. High-dose fish oil supplements may cause gastrointestinal discomfort and should be taken as directed.

Omega-3 fatty acids from fish are a valuable component of a healthy diet and are known for their potential health benefits. They are commonly consumed by incorporating fatty fish into the diet or through fish oil supplements. If you have specific health concerns or dietary requirements, consult a healthcare provider or registered dietitian for personalized guidance on omega-3 intake.

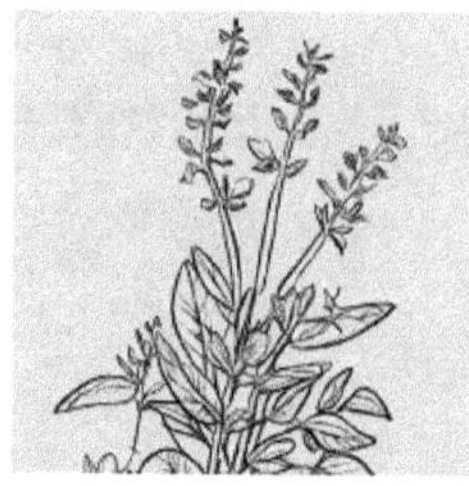

Oregano oil, derived from the leaves of the oregano plant (Origanum vulgare), is a popular herbal remedy known for its potential health benefits. It is often used as a dietary supplement or in aromatherapy. Here is a detailed overview of oregano oil, including its historical use, visual identification, medicinal properties, precautions, and potential health benefits.

Historical Use: Oregano has a long history of culinary and medicinal use, dating back to ancient Greece. Oregano oil has been used traditionally to treat various health issues, including respiratory and digestive problems.

Visual Identification: Oregano plants can be recognized by the following characteristics: Small, aromatic green leaves. Clusters of pink or purple flowers. The leaves are the source of oregano oil.

Medicinal Properties: Oregano oil is traditionally used for its potential health benefits, including Antibacterial and Antifungal: Oregano oil contains compounds like carvacrol and thymol, which have antibacterial and antifungal properties. Anti-Inflammatory: It is believed to have anti-inflammatory properties that can help reduce inflammation and pain. Antioxidant: Oregano oil is rich in antioxidants that help protect cells from oxidative damage.

Respiratory Health: It is often used to alleviate respiratory issues, such as colds, coughs, and bronchitis. Digestive Health: Oregano oil may support digestive health and help relieve issues like indigestion and gas.

Precautions: Oregano oil is potent and should be used with caution. It should not be applied directly to the skin or taken undiluted by mouth. It may cause skin irritation or allergic reactions in some individuals, so doing a patch test before topical use is advisable. Consult with a healthcare provider before using oregano oil supplements or extracts for specific health concerns, especially if you have underlying health conditions or are taking medications.

Oregano oil is a versatile herbal remedy known for its potential medicinal properties, particularly in relation to its antibacterial, antifungal, and anti-inflammatory effects. It is commonly used in aromatherapy and as a dietary supplement. Consult with a healthcare provider before using oregano oil for specific health concerns, especially if you have underlying health conditions or are taking medications.

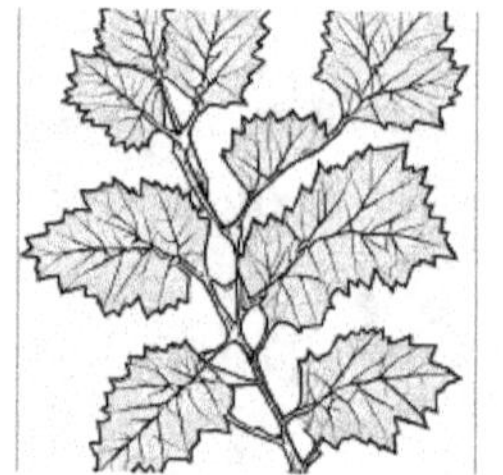 **Oregon grape (Mahonia aquifolium)** is a native North American plant known for its vibrant yellow flowers and purple-blue berries. It has a long history of use in traditional medicine, particularly among Indigenous peoples of North America. Oregon grapes are recognized for their potential medicinal properties and are often used as an herbal remedy. Here is a detailed overview of the Oregon grape, including its historical use, visual identification, growth conditions, medicinal properties, precautions, and potential health benefits.

Historical Use: Oregon grape has a history of use among various Native American tribes, who utilized it for its medicinal properties, including treating various ailments. It was also used as a dye for clothing and baskets.

Visual Identification: Oregon grape plants can be recognized by the following characteristics: Evergreen shrub with holly-like, pinnately compound leaves. Bright yellow, fragrant flowers in clusters. Small, purplish-blue berries that resemble grapes.

Growth Conditions: Oregon grapes are commonly found in the western regions of North America, particularly in forests and woodlands. It prefers well-drained, acidic soil and partial to full shade.

Medicinal Properties: Oregon grape is traditionally used for its potential health benefits, including Antibacterial: It contains berberine, a compound with antimicrobial properties that can help fight infections. Anti-Inflammatory: Oregon grapes are believed to have anti-inflammatory properties that can help reduce inflammation and pain. Digestive Health: It may support digestive health by improving liver and gallbladder function. Skin Health: Topical applications of Oregon grape alleviate skin conditions like psoriasis.

Precautions: Oregon grapes are considered safe when used as directed. However, it may cause mild side effects like stomach upset or skin irritation in some individuals. Consult with a healthcare provider before using Oregon grape supplements or extracts for specific health concerns, especially if you have underlying health conditions or are taking medications.

Oregon grape is a versatile plant known for its potential medicinal properties, particularly in relation to its antibacterial, anti-inflammatory, and digestive health benefits. It is commonly used in various forms, including herbal tinctures and topical ointments. Consult with a healthcare provider before using Oregon Grape for specific health concerns, especially if you have underlying health conditions or are taking medications.

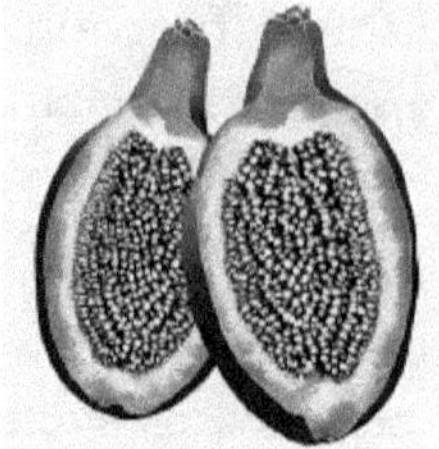

Papaya (Carica papaya) is a tropical fruit with a sweet taste and vibrant orange flesh. It is a delicious fruit and a popular natural remedy in traditional medicine. Papaya is known for its potential health benefits and versatile culinary uses. Here is a detailed overview of papaya, including its historical use, visual identification, growth conditions, nutritional properties, culinary uses, and potential health benefits:

Historical Use: use by Indigenous peoples for both its fruit and its medicinal properties. It was traditionally used to aid digestion and treat various health issues. Visual Identification: Papaya trees can be recognized by the following characteristics: Large, palm-like leaves. Single or multiple trunks or stems. Fruits are elongated and have orange to reddish-orange flesh.

Growth Conditions: Papaya trees thrive in tropical and subtropical climates with consistently warm temperatures. They require well-drained, fertile soil and regular watering.

Nutritional Properties: Papaya is highly nutritious and is a reliable source of vitamins. It is rich in vitamin C and provides a significant amount of vitamin A, particularly in the form of beta-carotene. Dietary Fiber: Papaya contains dietary fiber, which supports digestive health. Enzymes: They contain enzymes like papain, which can aid in digestion. Minerals: Papaya is a source of minerals such as potassium and magnesium.

Culinary Uses: Papaya is commonly used in various culinary applications, including Fresh consumption as a fruit. Smoothies and fruit salads. Salsas and chutneys, often paired with other tropical fruits and spices. Desserts like papaya ice cream or sorbet.

Potential Health Benefits: Papaya is associated with a wide range of potential health benefits, including Digestive Health. The enzyme papain in papaya can aid in digestion and may help alleviate digestive discomfort. Immune Support: The high vitamin C content may support the immune system. Antioxidant Properties: Papaya is rich in antioxidants that help protect cells from oxidative damage. Eye Health: The beta-carotene in papaya is beneficial for eye health and may reduce the risk of age-related macular degeneration.

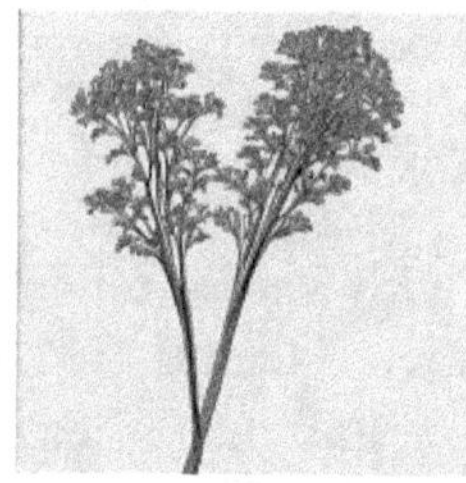

Parsley (Petroselinum crispum) is a versatile herb commonly used in cooking, known for its fresh, green flavor and its potential health benefits. It is a popular culinary herb garnish for various dishes. Here is a detailed overview of parsley, including its historical use, visual identification, growth conditions, culinary uses, nutritional properties, and potential health benefits.

Historical Use: Parsley has a long history of use in culinary and medicinal applications. It has been Greeks and Romans. In traditional medicine, parsley has been used to treat various ailments, including digestive issues.

Visual Identification: Parsley plants can be recognized by the following characteristics: Dark green, feather-like leaves. Small, greenish-yellow flowers in umbel-shaped clusters. A biennial herb, parsley typically grows as a rosette of leaves in its first year and produces flowers in the second year.

Growth Conditions: Parsley is a hardy herb that can be grown in various climates. It thrives in well-drained soil with good sunlight but can tolerate partial shade.

Culinary Uses: Parsley is a versatile herb used in various culinary applications, including Garnish: It is commonly used as a garnish to add color and flavor to dishes. Seasoning: Chopped parsley is often added to soups, stews, sauces, and salads for its fresh flavor. Tabouli: It is a key ingredient in the Middle Eastern salad called tabbouleh. Pesto: Parsley can be an alternative to basil in pesto recipes.

Nutritional Properties: Parsley is a nutrient-rich herb and a useful source of Vitamins. It is rich in vitamins, particularly vitamin K, vitamin C, and vitamin A. Dietary Fiber: Parsley contains dietary fiber, which is beneficial for digestive health. Minerals: It provides minerals like potassium, calcium, and iron. Antioxidants: Parsley is a source of antioxidants, which help protect cells from oxidative damage.

Potential Health Benefits: Parsley is associated with several potential health benefits, including Antioxidant Properties. The antioxidants in parsley may help protect against oxidative stress and associated health issues. Digestive Health: Parsley can support digestion and alleviate digestive discomfort. Immune Support: The high vitamin C content may support the immune system. Oral Health: Chewing parsley may help freshen your breath and promote oral health.

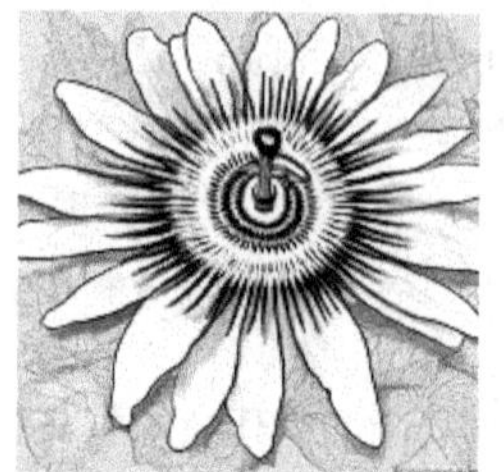

Passionflower (Passiflora incarnata) is a flowering plant known for its unique and intricate flowers. It is used both for its ornamental beauty and its potential medicinal properties.

Passionflower is commonly used as an herbal remedy to promote relaxation and reduce anxiety. Here is a detailed overview of passionflower, including its historical use, visual identification, growth conditions, medicinal properties, precautions, and potential health benefits:

Historical Use: Passionflower has a history of use by Native American tribes and later by European settlers for its calming and sedative properties. It has been used to alleviate anxiety, insomnia, and nervousness.

Visual Identification: Passionflower plants can be recognized by the following characteristics: Unique and exotic-looking flowers with intricate arrangements of petals and filaments. Vines with three-lobed leaves that may be green or with a tinge of purple. Round, fleshy fruit known as passionfruit, edible and sweet tasting.

Growth Conditions: Passionflower is a climbing vine that thrives in warm and tropical climates. It requires well-drained soil, good sunlight, and something to climb on, like a trellis or a tree.

Medicinal Properties: Passionflower is traditionally used for its potential health benefits, including Anxiety and Stress. It is used to alleviate symptoms of anxiety and stress, promoting relaxation and calmness. Sleep Aid: Passionflower is sometimes used as a natural remedy for insomnia and sleep disturbances. Anti-Inflammatory: It is believed to have anti-inflammatory properties. Antioxidant: Passionflower contains antioxidants that help protect cells from oxidative damage.

Precautions: Passionflower is considered safe when used as directed. However, it may cause mild side effects like dizziness or drowsiness in some individuals. It may interact with certain medications, particularly those that affect the central nervous system, so it is advisable to consult with a healthcare provider before using passionflower supplements for specific health concerns.

Passionflower is a unique plant known for its potential calming and sedative properties, particularly in relation to anxiety and sleep disturbances. It is commonly available in various forms, including herbal teas and supplements. Consult with a healthcare provider before using Passionflower for specific health concerns, especially if you have underlying health conditions or are taking medications.

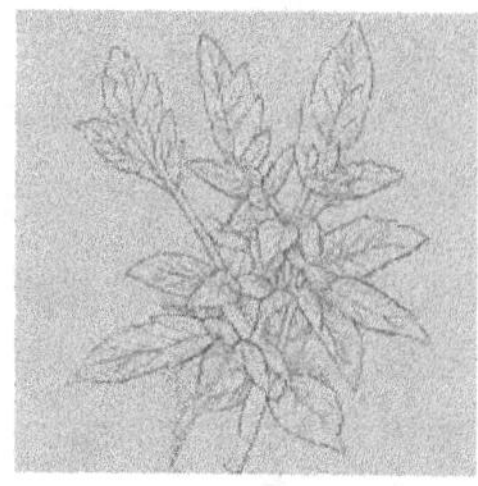

Peppermint (Mentha × piperita) is a is a popular and versatile herb known for its refreshing flavor and potential medicinal properties. It is widely used in culinary dishes, beverages, and herbal remedies. Peppermint is recognized for its soothing and cooling effects and offers a range of potential health benefits. Here is a detailed overview of peppermint, including its historical use, visual identification, growth conditions, culinary uses, medicinal properties, precautions, and potential health benefits.

Historical Use: Peppermint has a long history of use in both culinary and medicinal applications. It is a natural hybrid of water mint and spearmint and has been cultivated for thousands of   years.

Visual Identification: Peppermint plants can be recognized by the following characteristics: Opposite, lance-shaped leaves with serrated edges. Square stems. Small, purplish flowers in spikes.

Growth Conditions: Peppermint is a hardy herb that can be grown in various climates. It thrives in moist, well-drained soil and prefers partial to full sunlight. Culinary Uses: Peppermint is a versatile herb used in various culinary applications, including Flavoring. It is used to flavor beverages, such as tea and cocktails. Cooking: Peppermint leaves can be added to salads, desserts, and dishes for a refreshing taste. Baking: Peppermint extract or oil is used in baking to add minty flavor to cookies and sweets.

Medicinal Properties: Peppermint is traditionally used for potential health benefits, including.

Digestive Health. It can alleviate indigestion, gas, and bloating and may help relax the gastrointestinal tract muscles. Migraine Relief: Peppermint oil applied topically can help relieve headaches and migraines. Anti-Inflammatory: Peppermint is believed to have anti-inflammatory properties that can reduce inflammation and pain. Antispasmodic: It can help relieve muscle spasms and menstrual cramps. Breathing Aid: Peppermint can help open airways and ease congestion.

Precautions: Peppermint is considered safe when used as directed. However, it may cause mild side effects like heartburn or skin irritation in some individuals. It is important to use peppermint essential oil or extract cautiously, as they are highly concentrated and can be toxic if ingested in large quantities. Peppermint is a versatile herb known for its refreshing flavor and potential health benefits, particularly in relation to digestive health and soothing properties. It is commonly used in culinary and herbal reparations, making it a staple in many kitchens and households. Consult with a healthcare provider before using peppermint supplements or extracts for specific health concerns, especially if you have underlying health conditions or are taking medications.

Plant sterols, also known as phytosterols, are natural compounds found in plant cell membranes. They are structurally similar to cholesterol, a type of fat found in animal cells. Plant sterols have gained attention for their potential health benefits, particularly in reducing cholesterol levels and supporting heart health. Here is a detailed overview of plant sterols, including their sources, functions, and potential health benefits.

Sources: Plant sterols are naturally found in a wide range of plant-based foods, including vegetable, soybean, canola. and sunflower oil are useful sources of plant sterols. Nuts and Seeds: Almonds, walnuts, and flaxseeds contain plant sterols. Whole Grains: Whole grains like wheat germ and bran are rich in plant sterols.
Fruits and Vegetables: Certain fruits and vegetables, such as oranges, strawberries, and Brussels sprouts, contain moderate plant sterols.

Functions: Plant sterols play a role in plant cell structure and function, but their primary function in the human diet is their potential to reduce cholesterol absorption in the intestines. Plant sterols compete with dietary cholesterol for absorption, lowering cholesterol levels in the bloodstream.

Potential Health Benefits: Plant sterols have been studied for their potential health benefits, particularly in relation to heart health. Here are some benefits associated with plant sterols: Cholesterol Reduction: The consumption of plant sterols can lower levels of low-density lipoprotein (LDL) cholesterol, commonly called "bad" cholesterol. Lower LDL cholesterol levels are associated with a reduced risk of heart disease. Heart Health: Reducing LDL cholesterol levels is a key factor in preventing heart disease, making plant sterols a potentially valuable dietary component for individuals with heart disease.

Blood Pressure: Some studies suggest that plant sterols may also have a mild blood pressure-lowering effect, further contributing to heart health. Reduced Inflammation: Plant sterols may help reduce inflammation, a risk factor for heart disease.

It is important to note that the beneficial effects of plant sterols on cholesterol levels and heart health are more pronounced in individuals with elevated cholesterol levels. Plant sterols are often recommended as part of a heart-healthy diet for those with high cholesterol or at risk of heart disease. Plant sterols are available in various food products, including margarine, spreads, and fortified foods. These products are designed to provide convenient and standardized doses of plant sterols to help individuals manage their cholesterol levels. However, it is important to use plant sterol products as part of a balanced diet and under the guidance of a healthcare provider, especially if you have specific health concerns or are taking medications.

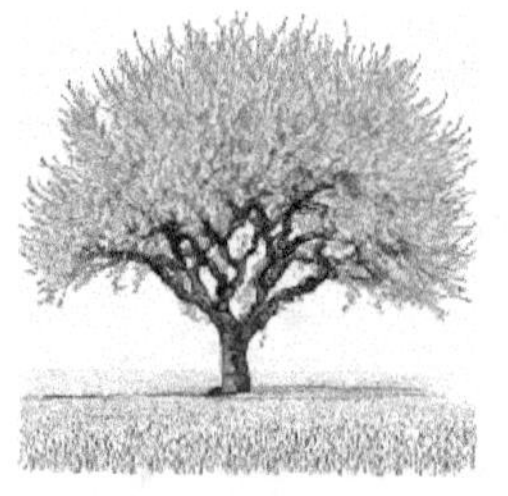

Plums (Prunus domestica) as Prunes. Prunes are dried plums, specifically from the European plum variety Prunus domestica. Prunes are known for their sweet and slightly tangy flavor, and they are often enjoyed as a healthy and convenient snack. They are also recognized for their potential health benefits, particularly in promoting digestive health. Here is a detailed overview of prunes, including their historical use, visual identification, nutritional properties, culinary uses, and potential health benefits.

Historical Use: Prunes have been cultivated for thousands of years and have a long history of use as a food and a natural remedy. They have been traditionally used to promote digestive health and alleviate constipation. Visual Identification: Prunes are dried plums and can be recognized by the following characteristics: Dark purple to blackish skin. Soft, wrinkled texture. Oval shape with a large pit in the center.

Nutritional Properties: Prunes are a nutrient-rich dried fruit are a useful source of dietary fiber. Prunes are high in dietary fiber, particularly soluble fiber, which supports digestive health. Vitamins and Minerals: They provide essential nutrients like vitamin K, A, potassium, and iron. Antioxidants: Prunes contain antioxidants that help protect cells from oxidative damage.

Culinary Uses: Prunes are enjoyed in various culinary applications, including Snacking. They are often eaten as a healthy and convenient snack. Baking: Prunes can be used as a natural sweetener and moisture enhancer in baked goods, such as muffins and cakes.

Potential Health Benefits: Prunes are associated with several potential health benefits, including Digestive Health. Prunes are well known for their natural laxative effect, promoting regular bowel movements, and preventing constipation.

Bone Health: The Prunes' vitamin K and potassium in prunes support bone health. Heart Health: Prunes may help reduce blood pressure and improve heart health due to their potassium content.
Antioxidant Properties: Prunes contain antioxidants that help protect cells from oxidative damage. It is important to incorporate prunes into a balanced diet for their potential health advantages, particularly for digestive health. If you have specific health concerns or dietary requirements, consult with a healthcare provider or a registered dietitian for personalized guidance on including prunes.

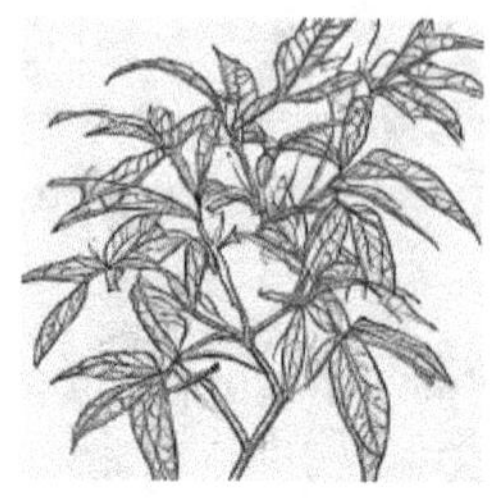

Pygeum (Prunus africana)

Pygeum, scientifically known as Prunus africana, is a tree native to certain regions of Africa. The extract from this tree's bark has been used for its potential medicinal properties, particularly in relation to prostate health. Pygeum is known for its historical use in traditional African medicine and is now a popular herbal supplement. Here is a detailed overview of Pygeum, including its historical use, visual identification, medicinal properties, precautions, and potential health benefits.

Historical Use: Pygeum bark has a long history of use in traditional African medicine for its potential health benefits, particularly in treating various urinary and prostate-related issues.

Visual Identification: The Pygeum tree can be recognized by the following characteristics: Large evergreen tree. Dark, smooth bark. Clusters of small, yellow to greenish-yellow flowers. Reddish-brown to black, oblong fruit.

Medicinal Properties: Pygeum bark extract is traditionally used for its potential health benefits, including Prostate Health. It is primarily used to alleviate symptoms of benign prostatic hyperplasia (BPH), a non-cancerous enlargement of the prostate gland that can cause urinary symptoms. Anti-Inflammatory: Pygeum is believed to have anti-inflammatory properties. Urinary Health: It may help improve urinary function by reducing urinary frequency and urgency associated with BPH.

Precautions: Pygeum is considered safe when used as directed. However, it may cause mild side effects like gastrointestinal discomfort in some individuals. Consult with a healthcare provider before using Pygeum supplements for specific health concerns, especially if you have underlying health conditions or are taking medications. Pygeum bark extract is a natural remedy with potential health benefits, particularly in relation to prostate health and alleviating BPH symptoms. It is commonly available in supplement form and is often recommended.

Quercetin is a flavonoid, a type of plant pigment found in various foods and plants. It is recognized for its potential health benefits and has gained attention for its antioxidant and anti-inflammatory properties. Here is a detailed overview of quercetin, including its sources, functions, and potential health benefits:

Sources: Quercetin is naturally present in many fruits, vegetables, and plant-based foods, including Onions. Red and yellow onions are particularly rich sources of quercetin. Apples: The skin of apples contains quercetin. Berries: Blueberries, cranberries, and blackberries are useful sources. Citrus Fruits: such as oranges and grapefruits contain quercetin. Leafy Greens: Spinach, kale, and lettuce are sources of quercetin. Tomatoes: Quercetin is found in the skin of tomatoes. Tea: Black and green tea contains quercetin.
Red Wine: Some red wines contain quercetin.

Functions: Quercetin is a potent antioxidant and anti-inflammatory compound. Its functions and potential health benefits include antioxidant: Quercetin helps protect cells from oxidative damage caused by free radicals. This may help reduce the risk of chronic diseases. Anti-Inflammatory: It has anti-inflammatory properties that can help reduce inflammation and related health issues. Immune Support: Quercetin is believed to support the immune system and may help in preventing or alleviating allergy symptoms.

Heart Health: It may support heart health by improving blood vessel function and reducing blood pressure. Cognitive Health: Quercetin may have neuroprotective properties and support cognitive health.

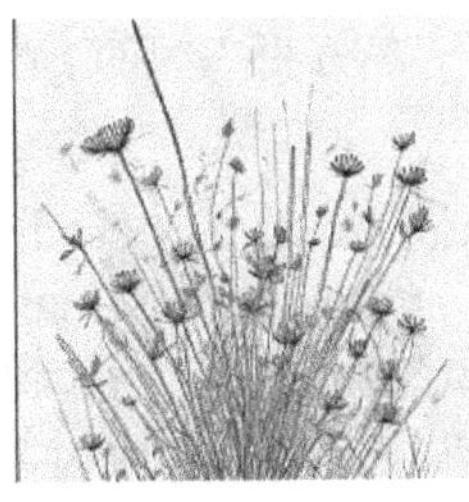

Red clover (Trifolium pratense) is a flowering plant that belongs to the legume family, and it is known for its potential medicinal properties. Red clover has a long history of use in traditional medicine and is recognized for its potential health benefits, particularly for women's health, and as a source of dietary isoflavones. Here is a detailed overview of red clover, including its historical use, visual identification, growth conditions, medicinal properties, precautions, and potential health benefits.

Historical Use: Red clover has been used in traditional medicine for centuries. It has been traditionally used to treat various ailments, including menopausal symptoms, respiratory conditions, skin disorders, and as a general tonic.

Visual Identification: Red clover plants can be recognized by the following characteristics: Trifoliate leaves with a characteristic white "V" mark on the leaflets. Red to pink, globe-shaped flower heads. Stems that can reach a height of 2 to 3 feet.

Growth Conditions: Red clover is a perennial plant commonly found in fields, meadows, and along roadsides. It prefers well-drained soil and can tolerate a range of soil types. It thrives in full to partial sunlight.

Medicinal Properties: Red clover is traditionally used for its potential health benefits, including isoflavones. Red clover is a source of dietary isoflavones, such as genistein and daidzein, which are phytoestrogens. These compounds may help alleviate menopausal symptoms in some women. Anti-Inflammatory: It is believed to have anti-inflammatory properties that can help reduce inflammation and related health issues. Cough and Respiratory Health: Red clover has been used to alleviate coughs and respiratory conditions. Skin Health: Topical applications of red clover extracts are used to treat skin disorders.

Precautions: Red clover is considered safe when used as directed. However, it may cause mild side effects like gastrointestinal discomfort in some individuals. It may interact with certain medications, so it is advisable to consult with a healthcare provider before using red clover supplements for specific health concerns, especially if you have underlying health conditions.

Red clover is a versatile plant known for its potential health benefits, particularly for women's health and as a source of dietary isoflavones. It is commonly available in various forms, including teas, tinctures, and dietary supplements. Consult with a healthcare provider before using red clover for specific health concerns, especially if you have underlying health conditions or are taking medications.

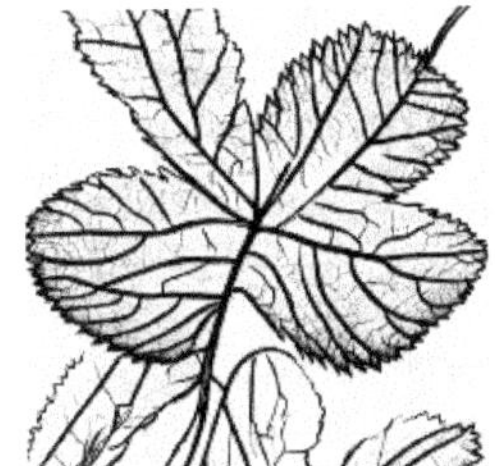 **Red raspberry leaf (Rubus idaeus)** is a well-known herbal remedy made from the leaves of the red raspberry plant. It is primarily recognized for its use in women's health and its potential benefits during pregnancy. Red raspberry leaf tea and supplements have been traditionally used for their potential health advantages. Here is a detailed overview of red raspberry leaf, including its historical use, visual identification, growth conditions, medicinal properties, precautions, and potential health benefits.

Historical Use: Red raspberry leaf has been used in traditional herbal medicine for centuries, particularly by Native American tribes. It is known for its potential benefits related to women's health, including during pregnancy and childbirth.

Visual Identification: Red raspberry plants can be recognized by the following characteristics: Deciduous shrubs with serrated, compound leaves. White to pale pink, five-petaled flowers. Red to yellowish-red aggregate fruits (raspberries)

Growth Conditions: Red raspberry plants are native to North America and are commonly found in temperate regions. They thrive in well-drained soil and are often found in woodland areas, along roadsides, and fields.

Medicinal Properties: Red raspberry leaf is traditionally used for potential health benefits, including Women's Health. It is commonly used to support women's reproductive health, particularly during pregnancy and labor. It may help tone the uterus and reduce the severity and duration of labor. Menstrual Health: Some women use red raspberry leaf to alleviate menstrual discomfort and heavy periods. Gastrointestinal Health: It is believed to have mild astringent properties to help soothe gastrointestinal discomfort. Antioxidant: Red raspberry leaf contains antioxidants, which help protect cells from oxidative damage.

Precautions: Red raspberry leaf is considered safe when used as directed. However, it is important to consult with a healthcare provider or a midwife before using it during pregnancy to ensure it is appropriate for your specific circumstances. It is advisable to use red raspberry leaf products that are specifically labeled for medicinal use, as the type and preparation can vary.

Red raspberry leaf is a widely recognized herbal remedy with potential health benefits, particularly for women's health, pregnancy, and labor. It is commonly available in the form of herbal teas and dietary supplements. Consult with a healthcare provider or a qualified midwife before using red raspberry leaf during pregnancy or for specific health concerns, especially if you have underlying health conditions or are taking medications.

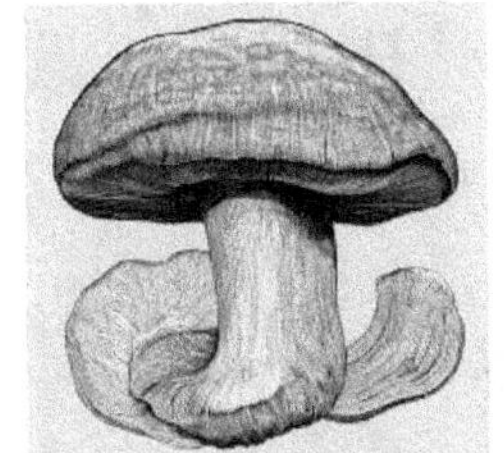 **Reishi mushroom (Ganoderma lucidum)**, also known as Lingzhi in traditional Chinese medicine, is a fungus that has been highly regarded for its potential medicinal properties for centuries. Reishi is recognized for its adaptogenic and immunomodulatory effects and is used in traditional medicine to support overall health and well-being. Here is a detailed overview of Reishi mushroom, including its historical use, visual identification, growth conditions, medicinal properties, precautions, and potential health benefits:

Historical Use: Reishi mushroom has a long history of use in traditional Chinese medicine and other traditional healing systems in Asia. It has been regarded as a symbol of longevity and vitality and is often referred to as the "Mushroom of Immortality."

Visual Identification: Reishi mushrooms can be recognized by the following characteristics. Shiny, kidney-shaped, or fan-shaped fruiting bodies. Typically, red to dark reddish-brown in color but can also be found in other colors like black, yellow, or green.
A shiny, lacquered appearance on the upper surface, with a white, porous underside.

Growth Conditions: Reishi mushrooms grow on hardwood trees, particularly oak and maple, but they can also be cultivated on sawdust or wood logs. They are typically found in East Asia but can be grown in other regions.

Medicinal Properties: Reishi mushrooms are traditionally used for their potential health benefits, including immune support.

Reishi is known for its immunomodulatory effects, helping to regulate and strengthen the immune system.

Stress and Adaptogenic Properties: Reishi is considered an adaptogen, helping the body adapt to stress and maintain balance.
Anti-Inflammatory: It is believed to have anti-inflammatory properties. Antioxidant: Reishi contains antioxidants that help protect cells from oxidative damage. Liver Health: Some traditional uses include supporting liver function and detoxification. Cardiovascular Health: It may help lower blood pressure and improve cholesterol levels.

Precautions: Reishi is considered safe when used as directed. However, it may cause mild side effects like stomach upset or skin rashes in some individuals. It may interact with certain medications or have blood-thinning effects, so it is advisable to consult with a healthcare provider before using Reishi supplements for specific health concerns, especially if you have underlying health conditions or are taking medications.

Reishi mushrooms are available in various forms, including capsules, extracts, and teas. They are often recommended as a dietary supplement for their potential health benefits, particularly in supporting immune function and promoting overall well-being.
Consult with a healthcare provider before using Reishi supplements for specific health concerns, especially if you have underlying health conditions or are taking medications.

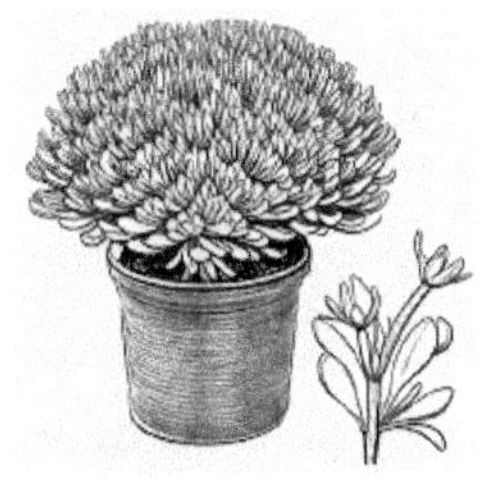

Rhodiola (Rhodiola rosea), also known as "golden root" or "Arctic root," is a medicinal herb with a long history of use in traditional medicine, particularly in Russia and Scandinavian countries. It is valued for its adaptogenic properties and potential health benefits related to stress and overall well-being. Here is a detailed overview of Rhodiola, including its historical use, visual identification, growth conditions, medicinal properties, precautions, and potential health benefits.

Historical Use: Rhodiola has been used in traditional medicine for centuries, particularly in Siberia and other parts of Russia, as well as in Scandinavian countries. It was traditionally used to combat stress, fatigue, and improve resilience.

Visual Identification: Rhodiola plants can be recognized by the following characteristics: Succulent, fleshy leaves with a bluish-green color. Small yellow flowers. Grows at high altitudes in cold and mountainous regions.

Growth Conditions: Rhodiola is typically found in high-altitude, cold, and mountainous regions of Europe, Asia, and North America. It thrives in rocky, well-drained soil and is adapted to harsh environmental conditions.

Medicinal Properties: Rhodiola is traditionally used for its potential health benefits. It is recognized as an adaptogen, which means it helps the body adapt to stress and maintain balance. Stress Reduction: Rhodiola is often used to combat stress, reduce fatigue, and improve mental and physical performance. Mood and Cognitive Health: It may positively affect mood, mental clarity, and cognitive function. Physical Endurance:

Rhodiola is believed to enhance physical endurance and exercise performance. Immune Support: It may support the immune system and help the body resist infections.

Precautions:
Rhodiola is considered safe when used as directed. However, it may cause mild side effects like insomnia, jitteriness, or dizziness in some individuals. It may interact with certain medications, so it is advisable to consult with a healthcare provider before using Rhodiola supplements for specific health concerns, especially if you have underlying health conditions or are taking medications. Rhodiola is commonly available as dietary supplements, including capsules and extracts. It is often recommended as a natural remedy for its potential health benefits, particularly in supporting stress management and promoting overall well-being. Consult with a healthcare provider before using Rhodiola supplements for specific health concerns, especially if you have underlying health conditions or are taking medications.

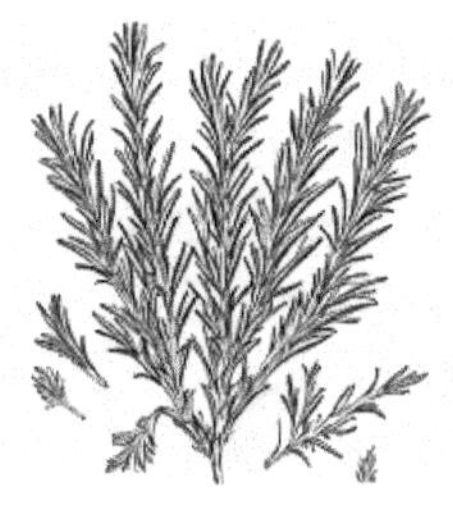 **Rosemary (Rosmarinus officinalis)** is a fragrant herb that is well-known for its culinary and medicinal uses. It is a versatile herb with a rich history of use in various cultures for its potential health benefits and aromatic qualities. Here is a detailed overview of rosemary, including its historical use, visual identification, growth conditions, culinary uses, medicinal properties, precautions, and potential health benefits:

Historical Use: Rosemary has been used for centuries in traditional medicine and culinary applications. It has a long history of being associated with memory and remembrance in various cultures. Visual Identification: Rosemary plants can be recognized by the following characteristics. Woody, evergreen shrub with needle-like leaves. Blue to purple flowers. Aromatic, resinous scent.

Growth Conditions: Rosemary is native to the Mediterranean region but can be grown in various climates. It prefers well-drained soil and full sunlight.

Culinary Uses: Rosemary is a popular culinary herb with a strong, aromatic flavor. It is used in a wide range of dishes, including Seasoning: Rosemary is used to flavor roasted meats, poultry, and potatoes. Baking: It is added to bread, focaccia, and other baked goods. Seasoned Oils and Vinegar: Rosemary-infused oils and vinegar are used in cooking. Marinades: It is included in marinades for grilling.

Medicinal Properties: Rosemary is traditionally used for its potential health benefits, including Cognitive Health. It has been associated with memory enhancement and mental clarity. Anti-Inflammatory: Rosemary is believed to have anti-inflammatory properties. Antioxidant: It contains antioxidants that help protect cells from oxidative damage. Digestive Health: Rosemary may support digestion and alleviate digestive discomfort.

Precautions: Rosemary is considered safe when used as a culinary herb. However, concentrated rosemary essential oil should be used with caution, as it can be toxic if ingested in large quantities. It may interact with certain medications, so consult with a healthcare provider before using rosemary supplements for specific health concerns, especially if you have underlying health conditions or are taking medications.

Rosemary is a versatile herb that is commonly used in cooking and for its potential health benefits, particularly in relation to cognitive health and antioxidant properties. It is a staple in many kitchens and households. Consult with a healthcare provider before using rosemary supplements for specific health concerns, especially if you have underlying health conditions or are taking medications.

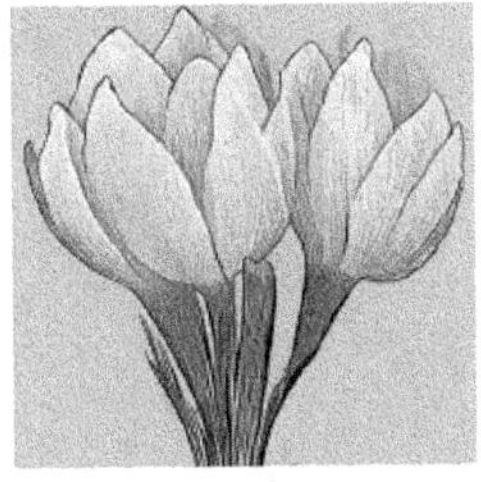

Saffron (Crocus sativus) is one of the world's most expensive and sought-after spices, known for its distinct flavor, aroma, and vibrant red-orange color. It is derived from the stigma (the female reproductive part) of the saffron crocus flower. Saffron has a rich history of use in culinary and traditional medicine practices and is valued for its unique properties. Here is a detailed overview of saffron, including its historical use, visual identification, growth conditions, culinary uses, medicinal properties, precautions, and potential health benefits.

Historical Use: Saffron has been used for thousands of years, with historical records dating back to ancient civilizations. It has been used in culinary dishes, perfumes, and traditional medicine. Saffron has been particularly valued in Persian, Indian, and Mediterranean cuisines.

Visual Identification: Saffron crocus flowers and saffron stigmas can be recognized by the following characteristics: Saffron crocus flowers are purple with three vivid crimson stigmas. The stigmas, which are the parts collected for saffron, are bright red-orange threads that are carefully separated from the rest of the flower.

Growth Conditions: The saffron crocus is a fall-blooming flower that thrives in regions with a Mediterranean climate. It prefers well-drained, loamy soil and full sunlight.

Culinary Uses: Saffron is a highly prized spice used in various culinary applications, including Flavoring. Saffron imparts a unique and distinct flavor to dishes, often described as floral, honey-like, and slightly bitter. Aroma: It adds a sweet and earthy aroma to foods. Color: Saffron gives a rich golden-yellow or orange color to dishes, such as paella and risotto. Beverages: It is used to flavor and color beverages like saffron tea.

Medicinal Properties: Saffron has been used in traditional medicine for its potential health benefits, including Mood Enhancement. Saffron may have mood-enhancing properties and is used to alleviate symptoms of mild to moderate depression. Antioxidant: It contains antioxidants that help protect cells from oxidative damage. Digestive Health: Saffron is believed to support digestion and alleviate digestive discomfort.

Precautions: Saffron is considered safe when used moderately as a spice in culinary dishes. However, saffron supplements should be used with caution and under the guidance of a healthcare provider, as excessive intake can be harmful. Consult with a healthcare provider before using saffron supplements for specific health concerns, especially if you have underlying health conditions or are taking medications. Saffron is a highly prized and versatile spice used in various culinary dishes and traditional medicine practices. It is known for its unique flavor, aroma, and color. When used responsibly, saffron can add a delightful and distinctive element to many recipes and offer potential health benefits.

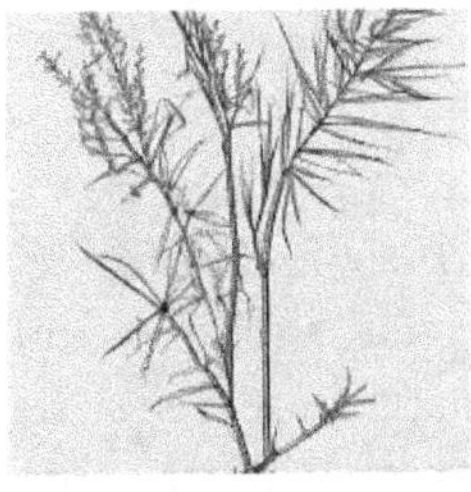

Senna is a group of flowering plants belonging to the Cassia genus, with several species, including Cassia acutifolia and Cassia angustifolia, commonly used for their laxative properties. Senna has a long history of use as a natural remedy to alleviate constipation and promote bowel movements. Here is a detailed overview of senna, including its historical use, visual identification, medicinal properties, precautions, and potential health benefits.

Historical Use: Senna has been used for centuries, dating back to ancient Egyptian and Arabian traditional medicine. It has been valued for its laxative properties and as a natural way to relieve constipation.

Visual Identification: Senna plants can be recognized by the following characteristics: Herbaceous plants with pinnate leaves. Yellow, butterfly-shaped flowers. Long, slender seed pods.

Medicinal Properties: Senna is traditionally used for its potential medicinal properties, including its strong laxative effect. It contains compounds called sennosides that stimulate the muscles in the intestines, promoting bowel movements.

Precautions: Senna should be used cautiously and only occasionally to relieve acute constipation. Prolonged or excessive use of senna can lead to various side effects, including diarrhea, abdominal cramps, electrolyte imbalances, and dependence on laxatives. It is vital to use under the guidance of a healthcare provider, particularly if you have underlying health conditions or are taking medications.

Long-term and frequent use of senna is not recommended and can lead to a condition known as "laxative dependency."

Senna is commonly available in various forms, including as herbal teas, capsules, tablets, and liquid extracts, and is often recommended as a short-term solution for constipation relief. It should be used cautiously and only for short-term relief of acute constipation. Consult with a healthcare provider before using Senna for specific health concerns, especially if you have underlying health conditions or are taking medications.

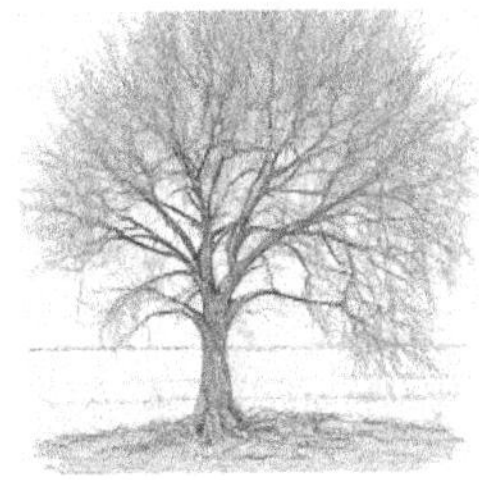

Slippery elm (Ulmus rubra) is a deciduous tree native to North America. It is known for its mucilaginous inner bark, which has been used in traditional herbal medicine for its potential soothing and healing properties. The inner bark of slippery elm contains mucilage, a gel-like substance that becomes slippery and soothing when mixed with water. Here is a detailed overview of slippery elm, including its historical use, visual identification, medicinal properties, precautions, and potential health benefits.

Historical Use: Slippery elm has a long history of use in traditional Native American medicine and was adopted by early European settlers in North America. It was used as a natural remedy for various health issues, particularly for soothing sore throats and digestive discomfort.

Visual Identification: Slippery elm trees can be recognized by the following characteristics: Deciduous trees with rough, reddish-brown bark. Leaves are elliptical with serrated edges and prominent veins. The inner bark is used for medicinal purposes and has a slippery, mucilaginous texture when mixed with water.

Medicinal Properties: Slippery elm is traditionally used for potential health benefits, including soothing sore throats. slippery elm lozenges or teas are often used to soothe the discomfort of sore throats and coughs.

Digestive Health: It may help alleviate digestive discomfort, including heartburn, gastritis, and diarrhea, by coating the digestive tract and reducing irritation. Skin Health: Some topical preparations with slippery elm may be used to soothe skin irritations and minor wounds.

Precautions:
Slippery elm is considered safe when used as directed, but individuals with known allergies to elm trees should avoid it. It may interfere with the absorption of certain medications, so it is advisable to consult with a healthcare provider before using slippery elm supplements for specific health concerns, especially if you have underlying health conditions or are taking medications. Slippery elm is commonly available in the form of lozenges, teas, and capsules and is often recommended as a natural remedy for soothing sore throats, digestive discomfort, and skin irritations. Consult with a healthcare provider before using Slippery Elm supplements for specific health concerns, especially if you have underlying health conditions or are taking medications.

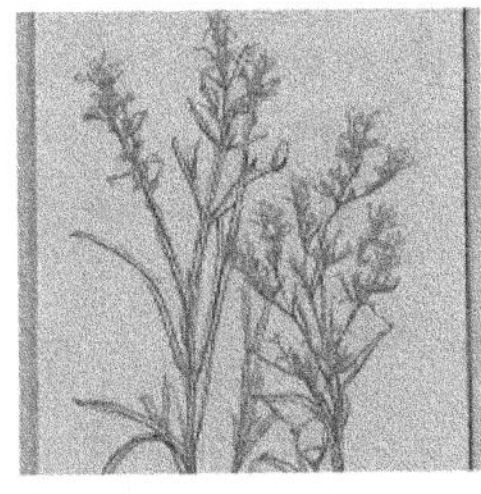

St. John's wort (Hypericum perforatum) is a flowering plant known for its potential medicinal properties, particularly for treating mood disorders and mild to moderate depression. It is a well-known herbal remedy with a history of use dating back to ancient times. Here is a detailed overview of St. John's wort, including its historical use, visual identification, medicinal properties, precautions, and potential health benefits.

Historical Use: St. John's wort has a long history of use in traditional medicine, dating back to the ancient Greeks and Romans. It was traditionally used to treat various ailments, including anxiety, wounds, and nerve pain. It is named after St. John the Baptist because it blooms around the time of the feast of St. John.

Visual Identification: St. John's wort plants can be recognized by the following characteristics: Perennial herb with bright yellow flowers with distinct black dots. Opposite, narrow leaves. Grows in various habitats, including meadows, fields, and along roadsides.

Medicinal Properties: St. John's wort is traditionally used for its potential health benefits, including Antidepressant Properties. It is primarily known for its potential to alleviate mild to moderate depression. It contains hypericin and hyperforin, compounds believed to play a role in its antidepressant effects. Anxiety Relief: St. John's wort may help reduce symptoms of anxiety. Anti-Inflammatory: It is believed to have anti-inflammatory properties.

Antiviral: St. John's wort has been used to treat certain viral infections, such as herpes. Wound Healing: Topical preparations with St. John's wort have been used to promote wound healing.

Precautions:
St. John's wort can interact with various medications, including birth control pills, blood-thinning medications, and antidepressants. It can affect their effectiveness and safety, so it is crucial to consult a healthcare provider before using St. John's wort if you are taking medications. It may cause side effects, including gastrointestinal discomfort, skin sensitivity to sunlight, and allergic reactions in some individuals. St. John's wort should not replace prescription medications for severe depression or other serious mental health conditions. St. John's wort is commonly available in the form of capsules, tablets, and liquid extracts and is often recommended as a natural remedy for mild to moderate depression and anxiety. Consult with a healthcare provider before using St. John's wort supplements, especially if you are taking medications or have underlying health conditions.

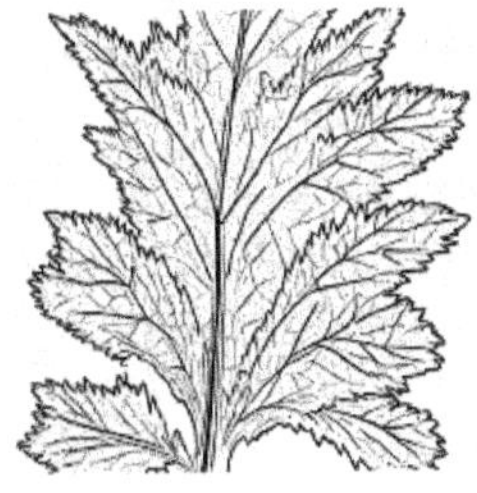 **Stinging nettle (Urtica dioica)** is an herbaceous plant well-known for its potential medicinal properties and often used in traditional herbal medicine. While the plant is covered in tiny hairs that can deliver a stinging sensation upon contact with the skin, it is valued for its various health benefits. Here is a detailed overview of stinging nettle, including its historical use, visual identification, growth conditions, culinary and medicinal uses, precautions, and potential health benefits.

Historical Use: Stinging nettle has a long history of use in traditional medicine, particularly in Europe and North America. It has been used for various purposes, including as a food source and for its potential medicinal properties.

Visual Identification: Stinging nettle plants can be recognized by the following characteristics: Toothed, opposite leaves with fine hairs that deliver a stinging sensation. Clusters of small, greenish, or yellowish flowers. Grows in moist, nutrient-rich soils and can reach heights of several feet.

Growth Conditions: Stinging nettle is commonly found in various regions, including Europe, North America, and Asia. It thrives in rich, moist soils, and it is often found in areas with partial shade.

Culinary Uses: Stinging nettle is a versatile plant used in culinary applications, especially when the leaves are cooked or steamed to remove the stinging hairs. It can be used in dishes such as soups, stews, and teas. It is valued for its potential nutritional benefits, as it is rich in vitamins, minerals, and antioxidants.

Medicinal Properties: Stinging nettle is traditionally used for its potential health benefits, including Anti-Inflammatory: It is believed to have anti-inflammatory properties and may help alleviate symptoms of conditions like arthritis. Diuretic: Stinging nettle promotes urination and may help with conditions like edema.

Allergy Relief: Some individuals use stinging nettle to alleviate symptoms of seasonal allergies. Prostate Health: It may have potential benefits for prostate health in men. Iron and Nutrient Content: Stinging nettle is a useful source of iron and other essential nutrients.

Precautions: While stinging nettle is considered safe when consumed as a food or herbal tea, it should be used cautiously as a supplement or for medicinal purposes. The stinging hairs on fresh nettle leaves can cause skin irritation, so they should be cooked or steamed to remove this effect It may interact with certain medications, so it is advisable to consult with a healthcare provider before using stinging nettle supplements for specific health concerns, especially if you have underlying health conditions.

Stinging nettle is commonly available in teas, supplements, and extracts and is often recommended as a natural remedy for various health concerns, particularly its anti-inflammatory and diuretic properties. Consult with a healthcare provider before using stinging nettle supplements for specific health concerns, especially if you have underlying health conditions or are taking medications.

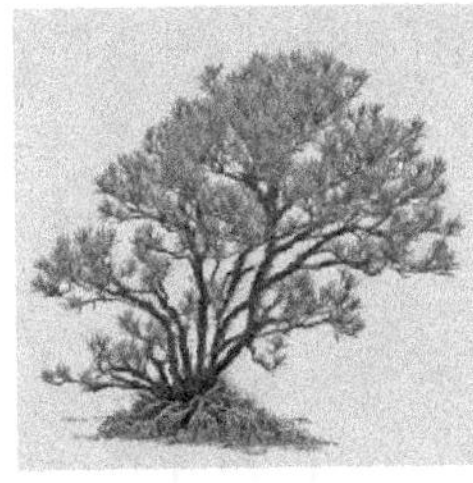

Tea tree oil (Melaleuca alternifolia) is an essential oil derived from the tea tree leaves, a native Australian plant. It is renowned for its potential medicinal and antiseptic properties and is commonly used in various topical applications. Here is a detailed overview of tea tree oil, including its historical use, visual identification, medicinal properties, precautions, and potential health benefits.

Historical Use: Tea tree oil has been used for centuries by Indigenous Australians, who crushed the leaves and applied them topically to treat various skin conditions. It gained recognition in modern times for its potential medicinal properties.

Visual Identification: Tea tree is a small tree or shrub with needle-like leaves and small, white, or purplish flowers. The essential oil is extracted from the leaves through steam distillation.

Medicinal Properties: Tea tree oil, including Antiseptic Properties, is traditionally used for its potential health benefits. It is valued for its antiseptic, antibacterial, and antifungal properties. It can treat minor cuts, wounds, and skin infections.

Skin Health: Tea tree oil is often applied topically to soothe skin conditions such as acne, athlete's foot, and nail fungus. Respiratory Health: It can be used for inhalation to relieve respiratory infections and congestion symptoms.

Oral Health: Tea tree oil is used in oral care products for its potential benefits in treating gum disease and bad breath. Insect Repellent: It is a natural insect repellent and can help alleviate itching from insect bites.

Precautions: Tea tree oil should always be used in diluted form when applied topically, as it can cause skin irritation or allergic reactions in some individuals when undiluted. It should not be ingested, as it can be toxic when taken internally. It may interact with certain medications, so it is advisable to consult with a healthcare provider before using tea tree oil for specific health concerns, especially if you have underlying health conditions.

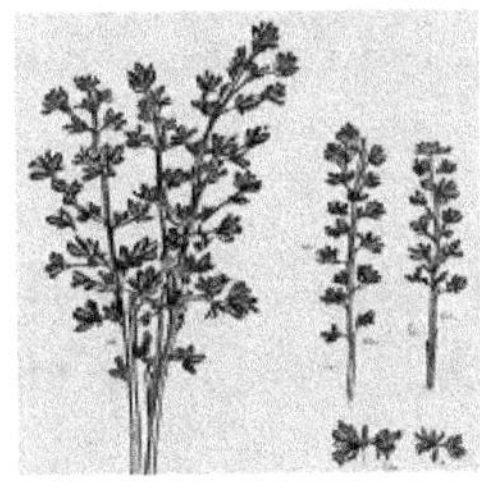

Thyme (Thymus vulgaris) is a popular herb and medicinal plant known for its culinary uses, aromatic properties, and potential health benefits. It is commonly used in various dishes and is also valued for its traditional medicinal properties. Here is a detailed overview of thyme, including its historical use, visual identification, culinary uses, medicinal properties, precautions, and potential health benefits.

Historical Use: Thyme has a long history of use, dating back to ancient Egyptian and Roman civilizations. It was used for its aromatic qualities, culinary applications, and potential medicinal benefits.

Visual Identification: Thyme plants can be recognized by the following characteristics: Small, woody, and perennial herb with tiny, fragrant leaves. It produces small white or pale pink flowers.
There are numerous varieties of thyme, each with slightly different appearances and flavors.

Culinary Uses: Thyme is a versatile culinary herb in many dishes, including Seasoning. It is used as a seasoning for meats, poultry, fish, and vegetables. Soups and Stews: Thyme is a common addition to soups, stews, and sauces. Baking: It can be used in bread, pizza dough, and various baked goods. Infusions: Thyme tea can be made for its flavor and potential health benefits.

Medicinal Properties: Thyme is traditionally used for its potential health benefits, including Antibacterial and Antifungal. Thyme contains compounds that may help combat bacteria and fungi. Anti-Inflammatory: It is believed to have anti-inflammatory properties. Cough Relief: Thyme is used in herbal remedies for coughs and respiratory congestion.

Digestive Health: It may support digestion and alleviate digestive discomfort. Antioxidant: Thyme contains antioxidants that help protect cells from oxidative damage.

Precautions: Thyme is considered safe when used as a culinary herb. However, thyme essential oil should be used with caution and always diluted, as it can be potent and may cause skin irritation when used undiluted. Thyme is not recommended for pregnant or breastfeeding women in medicinal doses, and it may interact with certain medications, so it is advisable to consult with a healthcare provider before using thyme supplements for specific health concerns, especially if you have underlying health conditions.

Thyme is readily available in dried and fresh forms for culinary use and as an essential oil or supplement for its potential health benefits. It is commonly used for its aromatic qualities and in various culinary dishes. Consult with a healthcare provider before using thyme supplements for specific health concerns, especially if you have underlying health conditions.

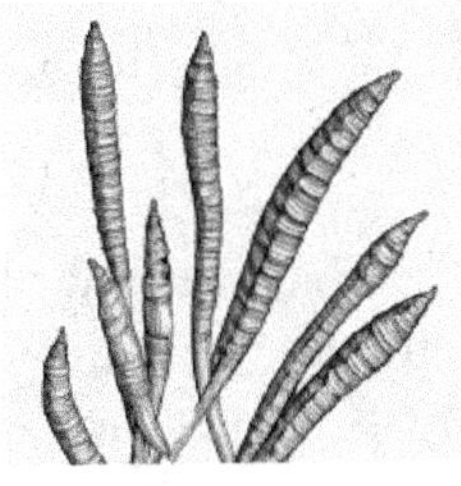 **Turmeric (Curcuma longa)** is a vibrant yellow spice and medicinal herb widely used in culinary and traditional medicine practices. It is renowned for its potential health benefits and is a key ingredient in many traditional cuisines. Here is a detailed overview of turmeric, including its historical use, visual identification, culinary uses, medicinal properties, precautions, and potential health benefits.

Historical Use: Turmeric has a long history of use in traditional medicine and culinary practices, dating back thousands of years, particularly in South Asia and India. It has been valued for its potential health benefits and vibrant color.

Visual Identification: Turmeric can be recognized by the following characteristics: Rhizomatous herb with tall leaves. Yellow or orange root or rhizome is used to make the spice.

Culinary Uses: Turmeric is a staple in many traditional cuisines and is used in many dishes, including Curry. It is a key ingredient in curry dishes. Seasoning: Turmeric flavors rice, soups, stews, and vegetable dishes. Beverages: Turmeric makes turmeric tea or "golden milk."

Medicinal Properties: Turmeric is traditionally used for its potential health benefits, including anti-inflammatory: It contains curcumin, a compound with anti-inflammatory properties that may help alleviate inflammation. Antioxidant: Turmeric is rich in antioxidants that protect cells from oxidative damage. Digestive Health: It is used to support digestion and alleviate digestive discomfort. Joint Health: Turmeric may have benefits for joint health and osteoarthritis. Liver Health: It is believed to support liver function.

Precautions: Turmeric is considered safe when used as a culinary spice. However, concentrated curcumin supplements should be used with caution and under the guidance of a healthcare provider, as they may interact with certain medications. In substantial amounts, turmeric may cause digestive discomfort in some individuals. Turmeric should be used with caution by individuals with gallbladder issues, as it can stimulate the gallbladder.

Turmeric is readily available in powder form for culinary use and as curcumin supplements for its potential health benefits. It is commonly used for its vibrant color and in various culinary dishes. Consult with a healthcare provider before using curcumin supplements for specific health concerns, especially if you have underlying health conditions or are taking medications.

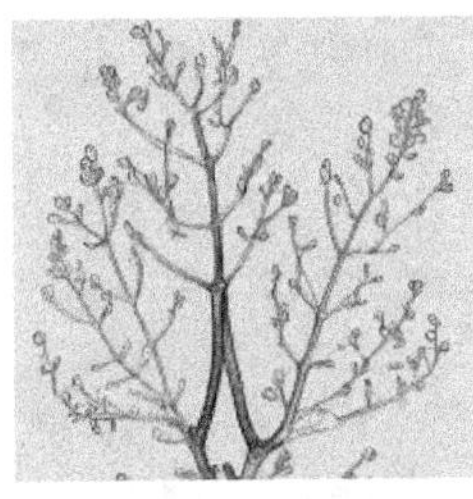

Uva Ursi (Arctostaphylos uva-ursi)

Uva Ursi, commonly known as bearberry, is a versatile and well-regarded medicinal plant native to North America. Uva Ursi has traditionally been employed for its role in promoting urinary tract health, its anti-inflammatory attributes, and its antioxidant properties.

Historical Use: Uva Ursi, also known as bearberry, has a history of traditional use by various Indigenous cultures, including Native Americans and indigenous peoples of Europe, for its potential medicinal properties. It has been used for urinary tract health and other health concerns.

Visual Identification: Uva Ursi can be visually identified by the following characteristics: Low-growing evergreen shrub with trailing stems. Small, leathery, shiny leaves that are green in the summer and turn reddish-brown in the winter. Pink or white bell-shaped flowers that bloom in early spring. Bright red berries that follow the flowers.

Medicinal Properties: Uva Ursi is traditionally used for its potential health benefits, including urinary tract health: Uva Ursi contains compounds, including arbutin, which may have mild diuretic and antiseptic properties, making it useful for promoting urinary tract health. Anti-Inflammatory: It may help reduce inflammation in the urinary tract. Antioxidant: Uva Ursi contains antioxidants that can help combat free radicals in the body.

Precautions: Uva Ursi is considered safe when used as directed for short-term purposes. It should not be used by pregnant or nursing women. Excessive or prolonged use of Uva Ursi can lead to liver damage and other adverse effects, so it should only be used under the guidance of a healthcare professional. Individuals with kidney or liver disease should avoid Uva Ursi. Uva Ursi should not be used by children under 12 years of age.

Potential Health Benefits: Urinary Tract Infections (UTIs): Uva Ursi is commonly used as a natural remedy to help prevent and manage UTIs due to its potential diuretic and antiseptic properties. It may help inhibit the growth of bacteria in the urinary tract. Anti-Inflammatory: It may help reduce inflammation in the urinary tract, providing relief for individuals with UTIs.
Antioxidant: The antioxidants in Uva Ursi may offer protection against oxidative stress.

Dosage: Uva Ursi is typically prepared as an infusion or tea. A common dosage is 1-2 teaspoons of dried Uva Ursi leaves steeped in hot water for 10-15 minutes. This infusion can be consumed up to three times a day. Consult with a healthcare provider or herbalist for personalized dosing recommendations, especially if using it for medicinal purposes.

It is essential to consult with a healthcare provider or herbalist before using Uva Ursi, especially if you have any underlying health conditions or are taking medications.

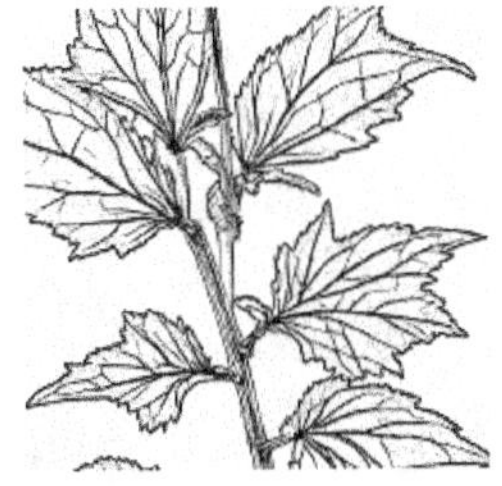 **Witch hazel (Hamamelis virginiana)** is a versatile and well-known medicinal plant native to North America. It is valued for its potential health benefits and is commonly used in skincare and traditional medicine. Here is a detailed overview of witch hazel, including its historical use, visual identification, medicinal properties, precautions, and potential health benefits.

Historical Use: Witch hazel has a long history of use by Native Americans for its medicinal properties. It was later adopted by European settlers in North America and has been used for various purposes, including wound healing and skincare.

Visual Identification: Witch hazel can be recognized by the following characteristics: Deciduous shrub or small tree with distinctive, forked, and twisted branches. Clusters of yellow, spidery flowers that bloom in the fall. Fruit capsules explode when mature, scattering seeds.

Medicinal Properties: Witch hazel is traditionally used for its potential health benefits, including Astringent. Witch hazel contains tannins that provide astringent properties, making it practical for toning and tightening the skin. Anti-Inflammatory: It may have anti-inflammatory properties and can help soothe irritated skin. Wound Healing: Witch hazel is used topically to help heal wounds and reduce itching and inflammation. Skincare: It is a common ingredient in skincare products like toners, cleansers, and ointments. Hemorrhoid Relief: Witch hazel is used for its soothing and astringent properties in managing hemorrhoid symptoms.

Precautions: Witch hazel is considered safe when used topically for its astringent and skin-soothing properties. While it is safe for most people, it may cause skin irritation in some individuals, so it is advisable to do a patch test before using it extensively.

Witch hazel products often contain alcohol, which can be drying, so individuals with dry or sensitive skin should use them with caution. Witch hazel is commonly available in the form of liquid extracts, toners, creams, and ointments and is often recommended for its skin-soothing and astringent properties. Consult with a healthcare provider before using witch hazel products, especially if you have underlying skin conditions or allergies.

Growing Table

This table provides general information about growing zones and seasons, but local conditions can affect plant growth. It is essential to consult local gardening resources and consider specific climate conditions for more precise planting and harvesting times.

Herb/Plant	Growing Zones	Season
Aloe Vera (Aloe barbadensis miller)	Zones 10-12	Year-round
Anise (Pimpinella anisum)	Zones 4-7	Spring to early summer
Astragalus (Astragalus membranaceus)	Zones 4-8	Spring
Bacopa (Bacopa monnieri)	Zones 9-11	Spring to summer
Bitter Melon (Momordica charantia)	Zones 10-12	Summer to fall

Black Cohosh (Actaea racemosa)	Zones 3-8	Late spring to early summer
Bladderwrack (Fucus vesiculosus)	Coastal regions	Year-round
Boswellia (Boswellia serrata)	Zones 10-12	Year-round
Buchu (Agathosma betulina)	Zones 7-10	Year-round
Butcher's Broom (Ruscus aculeatus)	Zones 6-9	Year-round
Butterbur (Petasites hybridus)	Zones 4-9	Spring
Calendula (Calendula officinalis)	Zones 2-11	Spring to fall
Caraway (Carum carvi)	Zones 4-7	Spring to summer

Cayenne Pepper (Capsicum annuum)	Zones 9-12	Year-round
Celery Seed (Apium graveolens)	Zones 2-10	Spring
Chamomile (Matricaria chamomilla)	Zones 3-9	Spring to early summer
Chasteberry (Vitex agnus-castus)	Zones 6-9	Summer
Chickweed (Stellaria media)	Zones 3-9	Spring to early summer
Comfrey (Symphytum officinale)	Zones 4-9	Spring to early summer
Cramp Bark (Viburnum opulus)	Zones 3-7	Late spring to early summer
Cranberry (Vaccinium	Zones 2-7	Fall

macrocarpon)		
Dandelion (Taraxacum officinale)	Zones 3-9	Spring to early summer
Dong Quai (Angelica sinensis)	Zones 5-9	Fall to early spring
Echinacea (Echinacea purpurea)	Zones 3-9	Summer to early fall
Eucalyptus (Eucalyptus globulus)	Zones 8-11	Year-round
Evening Primrose Oil (Oenothera biennis)	Zones 4-9	Spring to early summer
Fennel (Foeniculum vulgare)	Zones 4-9	Spring to early summer
Garlic (Allium sativum)	Zones 3-8	Fall to early spring

Ginger (Zingiber officinale)	Zones 10-12	Year-round
Ginseng (Panax quinquefolius)	Zones 3-7	Fall
Goldenseal (Hydrastis canadensis)	Zones 4-8	Spring
Green Tea (Camellia sinensis)	Zones 7-9	Spring
Horsetail (Equisetum arvense)	Zones 3-11	Spring
Lavender (Lavandula angustifolia)	Zones 5-9	Summer
Lemon Balm (Melissa officinalis)	Zones 4-9	Summer
Licorice (Glycyrrhiza glabra)	Zones 6-8	Late summer

Marshmallow Root (Althaea officinalis)	Zones 3-9	Summer
Mulberry (Morus spp.)	Zones 5-10	Summer to early fall
Mullein (Verbascum thapsus)	Zones 3-9	Spring to early summer
Neem (Azadirachta indica)	Zones 10-12	Year-round
Nettle (Urtica dioica)	Zones 3-10	Spring to early summer
Oats (Avena sativa)	Zones 2-11	Spring
Oregano Oil (Origanum vulgare)	Zones 5-10	Summer
Oregon Grape (Mahonia aquifolium)	Zones 5-9	Late winter to early spring

Papaya (Carica papaya)	Zones 10-12	Year-round
Parsley (Petroselinum crispum)	Zones 5-9	Spring to early summer
Passionflower (Passiflora incarnata)	Zones 6-9	Summer
Peppermint (Mentha × piperita)	Zones 3-11	Summer
Red Clover (Trifolium pratense)	Zones 3-8	Spring to early summer
Red Raspberry Leaf (Rubus idaeus)	Zones 3-8	Spring to early summer
Rhodiola (Rhodiola rosea)	Zones 1-4	Late spring to early summer
Rosemary (Rosmarinus officinalis)	Zones 7-10	Year-round

Saffron (Crocus sativus)	Zones 6-8	Fall to early winter
Slippery Elm (Ulmus rubra)	Zones 3-9	Spring to early summer
St. John's Wort (Hypericum perforatum)	Zones 5-8	Summer
Stinging Nettle (Urtica dioica)	Zones 3-10	Spring to early summer
Thyme (Thymus vulgaris)	Zones 4-9	Spring to early summer
Turmeric (Curcuma longa)	Zones 10-12	Year-round
Uva Ursi (Arctostaphylos uva-ursi)	Zones 2-7	Year-round
Witch Hazel (Hamamelis virginiana)	Zones 3-9	Late fall to early spring

Crafting Natural Remedies from Plants

In this chapter, we will explore various methods for creating natural remedies using plants. You will discover how to make balms, baths, gummies, infusions, oils, pills, poultices, presses, salves, syrups, and teas. These methods allow you to harness the healing power of plants and use them to address a wide range of health concerns.

Balms

Balms are semi-solid mixtures that combine plant extracts with fats or waxes. They are often used topically for their soothing and healing properties. To create a plant-based balm, Start with a base, such as beeswax or coconut oil, and melt it over low heat. Add your desired plant extracts, like chamomile, calendula, or lavender. These extracts can be in the form of essential oils or infused oils. Mix well, pour the mixture into containers, and let it cool and solidify. Balms can be used for skin irritations, minor burns, and dry skin.

Baths

Baths infused with plant materials can provide relaxation and relief from various ailments. Here is how to make a plant-based bath: Fill a muslin bag or a large tea ball with dried herbs, such as chamomile, lavender, or Epsom salt, and hang it under the running bathwater. Allow the water to circulate through the bag, infusing the bath with the plant's properties. Soak in the tub for a relaxing and therapeutic experience. Plant-based baths can help reduce stress, muscle relaxation, and skin conditions.

Gummies

Gummies are a delightful way to consume plant-based remedies, especially for children or those with trouble with other forms. To make plant-based gummies: Create a robust herbal tea infusion using dried plant materials like elderberries or echinacea.
Mix the tea with a gelling agent like agar or gelatin (for non-vegetarian gummies). Pour the mixture into gummy molds and let them set in the refrigerator. Plant-based gummies can support the immune system, improve sleep, or provide essential nutrients.

Infusions

Infusions are simple herbal teas created by steeping plant materials in hot water. To make a plant-based infusion, Boil water and pour it over dried herbs or plant parts, such as leaves, flowers, or roots. Cover the container and allow the herbs to steep for 10-15 minutes or longer for a more potent infusion. Strain the plant material and enjoy your herbal infusion. Infusions are a gentle way to consume plant remedies and can address various issues, including relaxation, digestion, and immune support.

Oils

Oils infused with plant extracts are ideal for massages and topical applications. To create a plant-based oil, Choose a carrier oil, like olive or coconut oil, and add dried herbs or plant parts to a glass jar. Seal the jar and place it in a warm, sunny spot for 1-2 weeks to allow the oil to infuse. Strain the oil to remove plant material and transfer it to a dark glass bottle for storage. Plant-based oils can be used for massaging skin conditions and as a base for salves and balms.

Pills

Pills or capsules are convenient for those who prefer a precise and tasteless way to consume plant remedies. To make plant-based pills: Create a fine powder from dried herbs or plant materials using a coffee grinder or mortar and pestle. Purchase empty capsules, which can be filled with the herbal powder. Cap the filled capsules and store them in a cool, dry place. Plant-based pills are commonly used for herbal supplements, such as turmeric or ginkgo biloba.

Poultices

Poultices are moist, plant-based preparations applied directly to the skin to address localized issues. To make a plant-based poultice, Crush or mash fresh or dried plant material, such as plantain leaves, comfrey, or calendula flowers. Add a small amount of warm water to create a paste. Apply the paste directly to the affected area, cover it with a cloth or bandage, and leave it on for a period of time. Poultices are effective for soothing insect bites, minor wounds, and skin irritations.

Presses

Presses or compresses are like poultices but often involve applying infused plant materials or oils to a cloth or bandage. To make a plant-based press, Infuse a cloth with a plant-based oil or herbal infusion. Apply the infused cloth to the affected area. Secure it in place with a bandage or gauze. Presses are used for various conditions, such as sprains, muscle soreness, and minor injuries.

Salves

Salves are semi-solid mixtures that blend plant extracts with oils and waxes for topical use. To make a plant-based salve: Melt a base like beeswax and combine it with plant-based infused oil. Add any desired essential oils for fragrance or additional properties. Pour the mixture into containers and allow it to cool and solidify. Salves are useful for skin conditions, wounds, and muscle soreness.

Syrups

Syrups offer a tasty way to consume plant-based remedies, especially for respiratory and immune support. To make a plant-based syrup: Create a strong herbal infusion or decoction using plant materials like elderberries or thyme. Strain the liquid and mix it with honey or another sweetener to create syrup. Store the syrup in a glass bottle in the refrigerator. Syrups can help soothe coughs, support the immune system, or provide relief from respiratory conditions.

Teas

Teas are one of the most accessible ways to enjoy plant-based remedies. To create a plant-based tea: Boil water and pour it over dried herbs or plant parts in a teapot or cup. Cover and allow the herbs to steep for the recommended time, typically 10-15 minutes. Strain and enjoy your herbal tea. Teas can address various health items - digestion, relaxation, and sleep.

Natural Recipes for Health

Peppermint Tea for Digestion:

Ingredients: 1 tbsp dried peppermint leaves, 1 cup boiling water Preparation: Steep peppermint leaves in boiling water for 10 minutes, strain, and drink. Recommended Dosage: 1-2 cups a day.

Interactions: May interact with medications that affect the liver's ability to metabolize drugs. Adverse Reactions: Rare, but in some cases, it can cause heartburn or allergic reactions.

Ginger Turmeric Immune Boosting Tea:

Ingredients: 1-inch piece of fresh ginger, 1 tsp ground turmeric, 1 cup hot water Preparation: Grate ginger into a cup, add turmeric and hot water. Let it steep for 5 minutes. Recommended Dosage: 1-2 cups daily. Interactions: May interact with blood-thinning medications or drugs that affect blood sugar. Adverse Reactions: Safe, but excessive consumption can lead to gastrointestinal issues.

Garlic Honey Infusion for Colds:

Ingredients: 2-3 garlic cloves, crushed, 1/2 cup honey Preparation: Mix garlic and honey. Take 1 tsp daily to boost the immune system. Interactions: May interact with blood-thinning medications and some antibiotics. Adverse Reactions: Garlic may cause digestive issues and skin rashes in some individuals.

Elderberry Syrup for Cold and Flu:

Ingredients: 1 cup fresh elderberries, 1 cup water, 1 cup honey Preparation: Simmer elderberries and water, mash, and strain. Mix with honey. Recommended Dosage: 1 tsp daily. Interactions: Rarely, it may interact with certain medications. Adverse Reactions: Safe but can cause digestive upset in some people.

Chamomile Salve for Skin Irritations:

Ingredients: 1 cup chamomile flowers, 1 cup olive oil Preparation: Infuse chamomile in olive oil for 2 weeks, then strain. Apply to irritated skin. Interactions: Safe when used topically.
Adverse Reactions: Rare, but it can cause allergic skin reactions in some individuals.

Chaga Mushroom Tea for Antioxidants:

Ingredients: 1 tbsp dried Chaga mushroom, 1 cup hot water
Preparation: Steep Chaga mushroom in hot water for 10 minutes.
Recommended Dosage: 1 cup daily. Interactions: Safe but consult with a healthcare professional if you are taking medications.
Adverse Reactions: Rare, but some individuals may experience mild digestive upset.

Calendula Tincture for Wound Healing:

Ingredients: 1 cup dried calendula petals, 1 cup vodka
Preparation: Combine ingredients in a glass jar, let sit for 4-6 weeks, then strain. Apply to wounds as needed. Interactions: Typically, safe for external use. Adverse Reactions: Rare, but skin irritation or allergy can occur.

Lavender Bath Salts for Relaxation:

Ingredients: 1 cup Epsom salts, 10 drops lavender essential oil
Preparation: Mix the ingredients and add to a warm bath. Interactions: Safe for topical use. Adverse Reactions: Rare, but skin irritation or allergy can occur.

Aloe Vera Gel for Sunburn:

Ingredients: Fresh aloe vera gel from the plant Preparation: Apply a thin layer of aloe vera gel to the sunburned area as needed.
Interactions: Rare but may interact with certain medications if ingested. Adverse Reactions: Safe when used topically, but some individuals may experience skin irritation.

Valerian Root Sleep Tea:

Ingredients: 1 tsp dried valerian root, 1 cup hot water Preparation: Steep valerian root in hot water for 10 minutes. Recommended Dosage: 1 cup before bedtime. Interactions: May interact with sedative medications. Adverse Reactions: Rare, but it can cause headaches, dizziness, and digestive upset in some individuals.

Turmeric Paste for Joint Pain:

Ingredients: 1/2 cup turmeric powder, 1 cup water Preparation: Mix turmeric and water to form a paste. Apply to sore joints. Interactions: May interact with blood-thinning medications. Adverse Reactions: Safe but can cause digestive issues in high doses.

Nettle Leaf Infusion for Allergies:

Ingredients: 1 tbsp dried nettle leaves, 1 cup hot water Preparation: Steep nettle leaves in hot water for 10 minutes. Recommended Dosage: 1 cup daily. Interactions: Safe but consult a healthcare professional if you have underlying health conditions.

Cayenne Pepper Salve for Muscle Pain:

Ingredients: 2 tbsp cayenne pepper, 1/2 cup olive oil Preparation: Mix cayenne pepper and olive oil, then apply to sore muscles. Interactions: Safe for topical use. Adverse Reactions: Rare, but it can cause a warming or tingling sensation.

Ginkgo Biloba Memory Tonic:

Ingredients: 1 tsp ginkgo biloba leaves, 1 cup hot water Preparation: Steep ginkgo leaves in hot water for 10 minutes. Recommended Dosage: 1 cup daily. Interactions: May interact with blood-thinning medications. Adverse Reactions: Safe but can cause headaches or digestive upset in some individuals.

St. John's Wort Oil for Nerve Pain:

Ingredients: St. John's Wort flowers, Olive oil Preparation: Infuse the flowers in olive oil for 2-6 weeks, then strain. Apply to affected areas. Interactions: Safe for external use. Adverse Reactions: Rare, but skin irritation or allergy can occur.

Reishi Mushroom Soup for Immunity:

Ingredients: 1 Reishi mushroom, Vegetable broth Preparation: Slice and simmer the Reishi mushroom in vegetable broth. Consume as a soup. Interactions: Safe but consult with a healthcare professional if you have specific concerns. Adverse Reactions: Rare, but some individuals may experience mild digestive upset.

Mullein Leaf Respiratory Tincture:

Ingredients: 1/4 cup dried mullein leaves, 1/2 cup brandy or vodka Preparation: Combine ingredients, let sit for 4-6 weeks, then strain. Take as needed for respiratory relief. Interactions: Safe but consult with a healthcare professional if you have specific respiratory conditions. Dandelion Root Coffee for Liver Health: Ingredients: Dandelion roots, Roasted chicory root Preparation: Roast and grind dandelion and chicory roots. Brew like coffee.

Interactions: Safe but consult a healthcare professional if you have a liver condition. It can rarely cause mild digestive upset in some individuals.

Lemon Balm Stress-Relief Tea:

Ingredients: 1 tbsp dried lemon balm leaves, 1 cup hot water Preparation: Steep lemon balm leaves in hot water for 10 minutes.

Recommended Dosage: 1-2 cups a day. Interactions: Safe but consult with a healthcare professional if you have specific concerns. Adverse Reactions: Rare, but in some cases, it can cause mild drowsiness.

Ashwagandha Elixir for Stress:

Ingredients: 1 tsp ashwagandha powder, 1 cup warm milk, Honey (optional) Preparation: Mix ashwagandha powder with warm milk. Add honey if desired. Recommended Dosage: 1 cup before bedtime. Interactions: May interact with certain medications, especially sedatives.

Fennel Seed Digestive Tea:

Ingredients: 1 tsp fennel seeds, 1 cup hot water Preparation: Steep fennel seeds in hot water for 10 minutes. Recommended Dosage: 1-2 cups a day. Interactions: Safe but consult with a healthcare professional if you have specific concerns. Adverse Reactions: Rare, but in some cases, it can cause mild digestive upset.

Milk Thistle Liver Detox Tincture:

Ingredients: 1/4 cup milk thistle seeds, 1/2 cup vodka
Preparation: Combine ingredients, let sit for 4-6 weeks, then strain. Take as needed for liver support. Interactions: Safe but consult with a healthcare professional if you have liver conditions.
Adverse Reactions: Rare, but it can cause mild digestive upset in some individuals.

Cinnamon and Honey Face Mask:

Acne treatment, Exfoliation, Moisturizer and Antioxidant Properties. Ingredients: 1 tsp cinnamon powder, 1 tbsp honey
Preparation: Mix cinnamon and honey to create a paste. Apply to the face for 10-15 minutes. Interactions: Safe for topical use.

Lemon Verbena Relaxation Tea:

Ingredients: 1 tbsp dried lemon verbena leaves, 1 cup hot water
Preparation: Steep lemon verbena leaves in hot water for 10 minutes. Recommended Dosage: 1-2 cups a day. Interactions: Safe but consult with a healthcare professional if you have specific concerns. Adverse Reactions: Rare, but in some cases, it can cause mild drowsiness.

Burdock Root Detox Soup:

Ingredients: 1 cup burdock root, Vegetable broth Preparation: Slice and simmer burdock root in vegetable broth. Consume as a soup. Interactions: Safe but consult with a healthcare professional if you have specific concerns. Adverse Reactions: Rare, but some individuals may experience mild digestive upset.

Sage Gargle for Sore Throat:

Ingredients: 1 tbsp dried sage leaves, 1 cup hot water Preparation: Steep sage leaves in hot water for 10 minutes. Use as a gargle. Interactions: Safe for topical use. Adverse Reactions: Rare but swallowing sage gargle can lead to mild digestive upset.

Rosemary Hair Rinse:

Hair Growth, Scalp Health and Shine and Softness Ingredients: 2 tbsp dried rosemary leaves, 2 cups hot water Preparation: Steep rosemary leaves in hot water for 30 minutes. Use as a hair rinse. Interactions: Safe for topical use. Adverse Reactions: Rare, but some individuals may be sensitive to rosemary and experience mild skin irritation.

Coriander Seed Digestive Infusion:

Ingredients: 1 tsp coriander seeds, 1 cup hot water Preparation: Steep coriander seeds in hot water for 10 minutes. Recommended Dosage: 1-2 cups a day. Interactions: Safe but consult with a healthcare professional if you have specific concerns.
Adverse Reactions: Rare, but it can cause mild digestive upset in some individuals.

Licorice Root Tea for Cough and Sore Throat:

Ingredients: 1 tsp dried licorice root, 1 cup hot water Preparation: Steep licorice root in hot water for 10 minutes. Recommended Dosage: 1-2 cups a day. Interactions: May interact with certain medications, especially those affecting potassium levels. Adverse Reactions: Rare, but excessive use can lead to high blood pressure.

Basil and Lavender Stress-Relief Bath:

Ingredients: Handful of fresh basil leaves a handful of dried lavender flowers Preparation: Add basil and lavender to a warm bath for relaxation. Interactions: Safe for topical use. Adverse Reactions: Rare, but some individuals may be sensitive to lavender and experience skin irritation.

Mint and Eucalyptus Steam Inhalation:

Ingredients: Handful of fresh mint leaves, Eucalyptus essential oil, Boiling water. Preparation: Add mint leaves and a few drops of eucalyptus oil to a bowl of boiling water. Inhale the steam for congestion relief. Interactions: Safe for inhalation. Adverse Reactions: Rare, but some individuals may be sensitive to eucalyptus and experience respiratory irritation.

Catnip Tea for Anxiety and Insomnia:

Ingredients: 1 tbsp dried catnip leaves, 1 cup hot water Preparation: Steep catnip leaves in hot water for 10 minutes. Recommended Dosage: 1-2 cups a day. Interactions: Safe but consult with a healthcare professional if you have specific concerns.

Astragalus Root Immune-Boosting Soup:

Ingredients: 1-2 slices of astragalus root, Vegetable broth Preparation: Simmer astragalus root slices in vegetable broth. Consume as a soup. Interactions: Safe but consult with a healthcare professional if you have specific concerns. Adverse Reactions: Rare, but some individuals may experience mild digestive upset.

Peppermint Oil Headache Relief:

Ingredients: Peppermint essential oil, Carrier oil (e.g., coconut or almond oil) Preparation: Mix a few drops of peppermint oil with a carrier oil and apply to the temples for headache relief. Interactions: Safe for topical use. Adverse Reactions: Rare, but excessive use may lead to skin irritation.

Yarrow Wound Powder:

Wound Healing, Antiseptic and Anti-Inflammatory Ingredients: Dried yarrow leaves Preparation: Grind dried yarrow leaves into a fine powder and apply to wounds. Interactions: Safe for external use. Adverse Reactions: Rare, but some individuals may be sensitive to yarrow and experience skin irritation.

Horehound Cough Drops:

Ingredients: Horehound leaves, Honey Preparation: Mix horehound leaves with honey to form cough drops. Interactions: Safe for use but consult with a healthcare professional if you have specific concerns.
Adverse Reactions: Rare, but some individuals may experience mild digestive upset.

Oregano Oil Immune Support:

Ingredients: Oregano essential oil, Olive oil. Preparation: Mix a few drops of oregano oil with olive oil and take as directed for immune support. Interactions: Safe when used as directed. Adverse Reactions: Rare, but excessive use may lead to digestive upset.

Saw Palmetto Hair and Scalp Treatment:

For Scalp and Hair Health and Moisture Ingredients: Saw palmetto berries, Coconut oil Preparation: Infuse saw palmetto berries in coconut oil for a few weeks and use as a scalp treatment.
Interactions: Safe for topical use. Adverse Reactions: Rare, but some individuals may experience skin sensitivity.

Dandelion Root Detox Tea:

Ingredients: 1 tbsp dried dandelion root, 1 cup hot water Preparation: Steep dandelion root in hot water for 10 minutes. Recommended Dosage: 1-2 cups a day. Interactions: Safe but consult with a healthcare professional if you have liver or kidney condition. Adverse Reactions: Rare, but it can cause mild digestive upset in some individuals.

Hibiscus Flower Heart-Healthy Tea:

Ingredients: 1 tbsp dried hibiscus flowers, 1 cup hot water Preparation: Steep hibiscus flowers in hot water for 10 minutes. Recommended Dosage: 1-2 cups a day. Interactions: May interact with blood pressure medications. Adverse Reactions: Safe, but excessive use can lead to a reduction in blood pressure.

Echinacea Immune-Boosting Tincture:

Ingredients: 1/4 cup dried echinacea root, 1/2 cup vodka Preparation: Combine ingredients, let sit for 4-6 weeks, then strain. Take as needed for immune support. Interactions: Safe but may interact with certain medications.

Black Elderberry Gummies for Cold and Flu:

Ingredients: Black elderberry syrup, Gelatin Preparation: Mix black elderberry syrup with gelatin to create gummies. Consume as directed for cold and flu relief. Interactions: Safe when used as directed. Adverse Reactions: Rare, but excessive use may lead to digestive upset.

Rose Hip Syrup for Vitamin C Boost:

Ingredients: Dried rose hips, Water, Honey Preparation: Simmer dried rose hips in water, strain, and mix with honey. Take as a vitamin C supplement. Interactions: Safe but may interact with certain medications. Adverse Reactions: Safe, but excessive use can lead to digestive upset.

Arnica Salve for Bruises and Swelling:

Ingredients: Arnica flowers, Beeswax, Olive oil Preparation: Infuse arnica flowers in olive oil, mix with beeswax, and create a salve for bruises and swelling. Interactions: Safe for external use. Adverse Reactions: Rare, but excessive use can lead to skin irritation.

Ginger and Honey Throat Lozenges:

Ingredients: Fresh ginger, Honey Preparation: Grate fresh ginger and mix with honey to form throat lozenges. Interactions: Safe when used as directed. Adverse Reactions: Rare, but excessive use may lead to digestive upset.

Borage Oil for Skin Health:

Ingredients: Borage oil Preparation: Apply borage oil topically for skin health. Interactions: Safe for external use. Adverse Reactions: Rare, but some individuals may be sensitive to borage oil and experience skin irritation.

Chickweed Skin Salve:

For Skin Irritations, Moisturizer and Barrier Ingredients: Chickweed leaves, Olive oil, Beeswax. Preparation: Infuse chickweed leaves in olive oil, mix with beeswax, and create a salve for skin irritations. Interactions: Safe for external use. Adverse Reactions: Rare, but excessive use can lead to skin irritation.

Lemongrass Relaxation Tea:

Ingredients: 1 tbsp dried lemongrass, 1 cup hot water Preparation: Steep lemongrass in hot water for 10 minutes. Recommended Dosage: 1-2 cups a day. Interactions: Safe but consult with a healthcare professional if you have specific concerns. Adverse Reactions: Rare, but in some cases, it can cause mild drowsiness.

Marjoram and Lavender Sleep Pillow:

Ingredients: Dried marjoram and lavender flowers Preparation: Create a sleep pillow with dried herbs to promote restful sleep. Interactions: Safe for external use. Adverse Reactions: Rare, but some individuals may be sensitive to lavender and experience skin irritation.

Goldenrod Allergy Relief Tea:

Ingredients: 1 tbsp dried goldenrod leaves, 1 cup hot water Preparation: Steep goldenrod leaves in hot water for 10 minutes. Recommended Dosage: 1-2 cups a day. Interactions: Safe but consult with a healthcare professional if you have specific concerns. Adverse Reactions: Rare, but in some cases, it can cause mild digestive upset.

Resources

For more in-depth, specific, or medically precise information on herbal remedies, interactions, and adverse effects, I recommend consulting reputable sources and experts in the field. Here are some reliable resources that you can use for further information on herbal remedies:

"The Complete Medicinal Herbal" by Penelope Ody: A comprehensive guide to medicinal herbs, their uses, and preparations.

"The Herbal Medicine-Maker's Handbook" by James Green: This book provides information on making herbal remedies and tinctures.

National Center for Complementary and Integrative Health (NCCIH): The NCCIH provides information and research on complementary and alternative medicine, including herbs.

American Herbalists Guild (AHG): The AHG is a professional organization for herbalists and offers resources on herbal medicine.

United States Pharmacopeia (USP): USP provides quality standards for herbal supplements and information on their proper use.

Botanical Safety Handbook: This handbook, by the American Herbal Products Association (AHPA), offers safety information for various herbs and botanical products.

"The Essential Guide to Herbal Safety" by Simon Mills and Kerry Bone: This book provides comprehensive information on the safety of herbal remedies.

Consulting with a certified herbalist or naturopathic doctor: For personalized advice on herbal remedies and potential interactions, it is advisable to consult with a qualified practitioner.

Index